THE FIRST YEAR®

Rheumatoid Arthritis

An Essential Guide for the Newly Diagnosed

M.E.A. McNEIL has written for the *San Francisco Chronicle Magazine* and is the author of *The Magic Storysinger: A Tale from the Finnish Epic Kalevala*, which won the Aesop Accolade from the American Folklore Society. Her new block-print-illustrated book of Finnish myth, *A Mother's Story*, has just been published. She lives in San Anselmo, California.

THE COMPLETE FIRST YEAR® SERIES

FORTHCOMING

THE FIRST YEAR®

Rheumatoid Arthritis

An Essential Guide for the Newly Diagnosed

M.E.A. McNeil

Foreword by Kenneth E. Sack, MD

MARLOWE & COMPANY ■ NEW YORK

Published by
Marlowe & Company
An Imprint of Avalon Publishing Group Incorporated
245 West 17th Street, 11th Floor
New York, NY 10011

AVALON
publishing group incorporated

Library of Congress Cataloging-in-Publication Data
McNeil, M. E. A.
   The first year—rheumatoid arthritis : an essential guide for the
newly diagnosed / M.E.A. McNeil ; foreword by Kenneth Sack.
       p. cm.—(The complete first year's series)
   Includes bibliographical references and index.
   ISBN 1-56924-364-6 (pbk.)
   1. Rheumatoid arthritis. I. Title: Rheumatoid arthritis. II. Title.
III. First year series.
   RC933.M376 2006
   616.7'227—dc22

                                        2005030694

ISBN: 1-56924-364-6
ISBN 13: 978-1-56924-364-0

9 8 7 6 5 4 3 2

Designed by Pauline Neuwirth,
   Neuwirth and Associates, Inc.

Printed in the United States of America

THIS BOOK IS FOR MY HUSBAND,
JERRY DRAPER,
WHO HAS SEEN ME THROUGH.

Contents

Foreword

by Kenneth E. Sack, MD

A DIAGNOSIS of rheumatoid arthritis conjures up feelings of dread in much the same way as a diagnosis of cancer. With cancer, death seems the inevitable outcome; with rheumatoid arthritis—deformity and dependence. In each case, reality suggests otherwise. Many forms of cancer are curable or compatible with a long and productive life. Rheumatoid arthritis may have a benign course on its own; but even at its worst, it is amenable to many disease-altering treatments.

The world of medicine is evolving at mind-boggling speed. Scientific knowledge is expanding exponentially, and access to most of these advances is accessible to the public via the Internet. Despite all our successes, however, many of the issues confronting patients with chronic illness remain the same— What caused my disease? What will this illness do to me? Can I be treated safely? Can I still have a life?

When I first met Mea McNeil Draper, she was spending most of her days in pain and in a wheelchair. Her rheumatoid arthritis was responding poorly to conventional treatment, and her doctors had not given her any cause for optimism. Mea was not one to give up easily, and I supported that optimism.

Fortunately, we were beginning a study of one of the new biologic agents, etanercept, and Mea became one of our first patients. The rest, one might say, is history. This class of drugs soon became the standard of care for those who had failed traditional agents, and Mea left behind her wheelchair as well as her bleak prospects.

Mea's successes, however, are only partially the result of antirheumatic medications. Her indomitable spirit and inquisitive mind are at least equally responsible for her remarkable achievements in life. It is this same spirit and intelligence that pervades the chapters of her book. And who can better get at the heart of what it takes to cope with chronic illness than someone who's been there, and who's triumphed!

KENNETH E. SACK, MD is a Professor of Clinical Medicine and Director of Clinical Programs in Rheumatology at the University of California at San Francisco. He writes on a wide range of rheumatic diseases for medical journals, textbooks, and international forums. He is currently working on a comprehensive study of Sjogren's syndrome.

Introduction

I remember the exact moment when I was diagnosed with rheumatoid arthritis: the last appointment of the day, the nervous new doctor young enough to be my daughter, a definition read out of a medical text, hopeless words hanging in the waning light.

You will remember, too, but your story will not be the story of my diagnosis—so much has been learned since that day for me in 1993. Your story is a new story in a new era, and you have every reason to be hopeful.

Although we still do not know everything about RA, enough is known now for us to manage a satisfying life. More is understood about the immune system, and more is known about how it is influenced by the mind. We also know more about what roles exercise and nutrition play in that relationship. There is a whole new category of RA drugs specifically targeted on a molecular level.

I could regret the years of my life when I was very sick with RA, but I know better. They were dark, yes, but that time was more like an alchemical cauldron in which I was transformed for the better.

Lance Armstrong said that if he had to choose between the experiences of disease and winning the Tour de France, he'd choose disease; he says it's made him more human. Fortunately, we are not faced with a life-threatening illness, but we can still be changed by a reappraised, refocused life. This diagnosis motivates us to begin to do things we've always intended to do to take care of ourselves. It changes our angle of vision; it prompts us to educate ourselves and act on what we learn. It can bring families and real friends closer. It can be a catalyst for us to simplify our lives and let go of things that are not important.

You are not entering the same dark unknown that I entered, but you are still entering a new world. It could be the best thing that ever happened to you. Until your new program is well under way, you'll have to trust me on this.

We are ready, with this diagnosis, to sign up for the easy cure, reason be damned. We all want to escape like Houdini—presto, ta-da, free! Well, it's possible; the trick is to think just like Houdini. We know that his magic was based on careful scientific analysis resulting in a plan and a calm, centered mind to execute it. That is the magic you will learn in this book.

You'll hear terrifying stories about people with RA, and if you don't know better you can simmer up a good depression over them. There is no shortage of tales about those who are crippled and deformed or bloated by medication—hey, I am a crooked tree myself. When I was diagnosed, the information brochure had the word "arthritis" written in a trembling hand. Even now, you can't mention your diagnosis without hearing about someone's great-aunt who can't hold a pen—or worse. But these stories are not your story. Plug your ears and lash yourself to the mast as you sail by the Sirens' songs of woe. Sure, you can crash on the rocks, but you have better choices now. And keep in mind that the anxiety that these stories carry works against your purpose.

This is not an exercise of mind over matter or a suggestion that you ignore your own negative experience. It simply does not help to be stressed about the people who did not have access to all you are about to find out and do. You and I have other options, and they are not woven of wishful thinking; our new choices are based on hard science. You are on one of the first waves through.

This is the book I would like to have had when I was diagnosed. I believe that much if not all of the damage I have in my joints would not have taken place if I'd had these resources. Lucky you.

Although three-quarters of us with RA are women, as individuals we are not statistics; we are of any age or gender. So I would like to address "you" as the person I was when I was diagnosed—a frightened human trying to find a way through a confounding diagnosis.

This book is designed to educate, not to prescribe, for I am not a doctor. I am not even the designated splinter-puller in my family, so you can be sure that I do not dispense medical advice. I have, however, assimilated information available in popular books, medical texts, and clinical studies. I've prowled the medical library at the University of California at San Francisco and begged materials reserved for rheumatology interns. I have been guided in my own treatment by an extraordinary physician. I have selected what I think will be useful to you in a format that I hope you will read with ease. The spirit of this book comes from over a decade of pondering this disease and how to live with it. But you will soon see that there is no one answer, and your path will be your own.

The ingenious format of this book, not of my devising, follows the timeline for oiling fine wood—every day for a week, every week for a month, every month for a year. Chapters are divided into sections called Living, about adjusting to life with RA, and Learning, with science behind choices you may want to make. Even if you do little technical reading, you may find these parts more fascinating than daunting. You can refer to words in **boldface** in the glossary at the back of the book. I have assumed your intelligence and provided a depth of material here that is rarely treated in popular books on RA.

As I write today, I work a regular day, keep a family and home in somewhat reasonable balance, and enjoy a relatively symptom-free life. Some say that this is too much to hope for with a diagnosis of RA. I will tell you what I have learned, and you can decide for yourself. Please listen in and take what you can use.

The Immune Metaphor

Warning: this metaphor is dangerous to your health

When I was diagnosed with rheumatoid arthritis, I read that my body was "attacking itself," that I was "under siege" by my own system. I felt scared, confused, and guilty. After all, I knew what it meant to beat oneself up over a mistake, and this had to have been some mistake.

The archaic belief that illness is punishment for some wrong-doing, as foolish as we know it is, still casts a long shadow over the way we think. I could only conclude that I somehow brought this upon myself, this anarchy of the knees.

Stress is described as a physical response to feeling over-whelmed, out of control. What could be more stressful than the mind-numbing concept of helpless self-destruction? In fact, it's a useless notion, worse than useless, so let's begin by retooling the metaphor.

Metaphors can get stuck onto facts, so it's good to remember that when they are no longer relevant, they are dispensable. History is littered with discarded metaphors, and we can add this one to the heap—along with the horseless carriage, the king bee, and women as helpless flowers.

True, it's useful for texts to use a military metaphor for the normally functioning immune system. Nature is an equal opportunity employer; consider how quickly road kill is picked to the bone by every local microorganism once the immune defense ceases. So it is reassuring for us to have immune "patrols" and "soldiers" guarding against "invasion."

Those of us with RA, though, whose immune systems have gone beyond a protective function, have no need to extend that metaphor to the idea that we are hurting ourselves. Cells in the immune system, some of which live less than a day, perform simple functions in response to chemical signals. These cells have no brains, no emotions; they are not pathologically hell-bent on destruction.

I appreciate a good metaphor when I am trying to understand, say, how macrophages affect the synovium. It serves you and me just as well to think of the story this way: Our "cleaning" cells keep working after the task is finished, like the gardener I hired who weeded so well that he took out the flowers. It was an error of communication rather than any malicious intent on his part toward dahlias. With RA, we have too many improperly signaled immune cells doing what they have been programmed to do for our health. We have too much of a good thing.

Once I realized that I was not, in fact, at war with myself, I could take a deep breath and consider what to do. I didn't need to "beat" or "conquer" it, as shelves of books exhort me to do. There is no foreign invader (although there could be a trigger), only my own cells—cells that normally perform a healthy, curative function.

A fighting stance is a place of stress, and science is telling us that stress has a negative effect on the immune system. There is enough aggression in the world without internalizing it. If I have learned anything from being a parent, it is that forcing a situation only creates a push-pull. It's like the old Chinese woven finger tube—try to force your fingers out and you just get more stuck; relax and they come free.

If we are looking for a metaphor, perhaps dance will serve—our bodies are our partners, and we need to learn to take the lead. It is a lot easier to tango than to quell an insurrection.

You'll still hear about insurgency in your joints, but you and I can cross that image off our list of worries. It's all the same, of course, except how we think about it, and how we think about it is one of the most important keys to managing RA.

IN A SENTENCE:

> *Useful metaphors for RA are those that don't hold us at fault.*

learning

What Is Rheumatoid Arthritis?

ASKING "What is rheumatoid arthritis?" is like asking, "What is this thing called love?" Well, there's the textbook answer, and then there is how it is for me, and then again, there is what it is for you—which is what this book hopes to help you answer. Like love, RA can be transforming, and, it's fair to say, for better or for worse. The textbook answer is clear: "Rheumatoid arthritis is chronic, inflammatory autoimmune disease of the joint lining," but some definitions still roll downhill to end in the last century with a thud in "progressive and debilitating." Well, there are "fifty ways to leave your lover," and there are just as many ways for most of us to get out of that prognosis.

A hundred types of arthritis

"Arthritis" turns out to be a portmanteau word, commonly used to refer to the joint discomfort of any of a hundred or so diseases. Although there are shared symptoms of pain, stiffness, and often swelling of the joints, the similarities stop there. In general they fall into two categories:

Osteoarthritis—mechanical joint problems caused by wear
Inflammatory arthritis—including:
    infectious arthritis, which is not infecting but caused by a pathogen—
       like Lyme disease. (No type of arthritis is contagious.)
    systemic autoimmune disease, including rheumatoid arthritis, anky-
       losing spondylitis, lupus, gout, among others—diverse diseases.

Chances are, when you run into one of the forty million Americans who say that she, too, has arthritis, it will turn out to be osteoarthritis, the most common form. If you are booking the odds, there are three times as many women than men.

In osteoarthritis, the **cartilage**, which protects the ends of bones in the joints, wears away with use until bone rubs on bone. Osteoarthritis most often affects the fingers and weight-bearing joints—knees, hips, spine, and neck. Using the joints can cause inflammation in OA; conversely, in RA, movement can help inflammation subside. You may hear of people with any kind of arthritis who predict the weather from the pain in their joints, but I have yet to hear a report that I could ski on.

Rheumatoid arthritis is a relatively recent disease

Rheumatoid arthritis affects over two million Americans and over fifty million people worldwide. Like osteoarthritis, it is three times more common in women than in men. Onset of the disease is increasingly more common with age, peaking in the middle years. Heredity is a factor, together with environmental influences. (Look ahead to Months 4 and 5 to learn more.)

What appears to be evidence of rheumatoid arthritis was noted in skeletal remains of Native Americans from 4500 BCE found in what is now Tennessee. Apart from that, there is no evidence of the disease in ancient times. (The arthritis found in Egyptian mummies is osteoarthritis.)

The disease was not named until the mid-nineteenth century, when a London doctor chose, in the contemporary fashion for Greek labels on medical matters, *arthron*, meaning joint, and *itis*, inflammation. (Consider *inflammare*, the Latin verb meaning "to set on fire," if you want to torture yourself with etymology.) The Greek *rheuma* was added, meaning watery flow, to describe our particular squishy hinges.

Recorded cases from the nineteenth century up until people still living today show us well the devastating effects of the uncontrolled course of the disease. Pierre-Auguste Renoir, the renowned French impressionist, began to suffer symptoms of rheumatoid arthritis in 1882. Doctors prescribed enemas and fever medications—not much less effective than would be available for another half-century. His joint pain was so severe that his bed covers had to be tented over him. Over the next twenty years, he was carried to his easel every morning, where he continued painting with a brush wedged into his hands. He died at seventy-eight from pneumonia, a complication of advanced rheumatoid arthritis.

These are not the 'roids you're looking for

The autoimmune theory that holds true today was formulated in 1939 by an Australian researcher, and in 1941 rheumatoid arthritis was recognized as a distinct disorder. The modern American field of rheumatology was started a few years later.

The discoverers of the anti-inflammatory effects of steroid hormones in 1948 won a Nobel Prize. About the same time, the antibody known as the rheumatoid factor was isolated in the blood of some people with rheumatoid arthritis, and a diagnostic test was devised. (It is approximate; you can read more about it in Week 5.)

In the year 1955 a love-hate relationship began with a drug many with RA have known so well. Prednisone, a synthetic derivative of cortisone, was introduced and dispensed as a wonder drug—before its serious side effects became known.

We have only recently stepped out of the dark ages; the actress Viveca Lindfors died in 1995 of complications from rheumatoid arthritis—something that may become as rare as a death from smallpox for those diagnosed today. As for me, I am like a fish with legs, an anachronism with a foot in two worlds—quite literally in fact, with bone destruction halted by a new drug. (See Weeks 6 and 7 to learn more about drugs.)

So much for the requisite history lesson; now you belong to the RA club. (One member with a twisted sense of humor calls us RAbies.)

What are the symptoms?

Facts: Climate neither causes nor cures arthritis. We don't get it from cracking our knuckles. Apart from that, you are entering individual territory.

The disease does follow a general pattern: of the one hundred fifty joints in the body, there are rigid joints like those of the skull, joints with slight mobility like those of the spine, and free-moving joints, which are the sites of RA. There are seventy of these movable joints, called **synovial joints**, and it is usually the smaller ones that are involved. Beyond that, it is unlikely that your experience will be exactly like anyone else's.

A characteristic early complaint is joint stiffness upon waking, called the **gel phenomenon**, and it sometimes lasts for hours. The swelling is caused by the accumulation of fluid in inflamed tissues, and the fluid is gradually absorbed back into blood when joints start moving.

For me, it started with aching feet, but it can start in the joints of the fingers or wrists; any joint can be the first site. It can begin so gradually that it is hard to remember. That first sign is an inflammation of the joint lining, which causes a nagging ache. Sometimes a feeling of weakness or fatigue comes on before joint pain. More rarely, it can begin suddenly with many painfully swollen joints.

The amount of joint pain varies, as does an individual's tolerance for pain. Although it can be severe and constant for some, many have moderate pain that comes and goes.

Classic RA develops symmetrically; the same joint on both sides of the body is affected. Joints can be warm, swollen, tender, and sometimes red. Often, discomfort begins in one or two joints and spreads to many joints. Typically the fingers, hands, wrists, elbows, shoulders, knees, ankles, and feet are involved. The jaw and neck can also be affected. Involvement of larger joints in the hips is found more often in men. Fatigue, a common symptom, often descends in the afternoon. It is the body's reaction to substances released into bloodstream by activated immune cells. Some people have flu-like symptoms, a low-grade fever, a feeling described as "sick all over." Symptoms may appear simultaneously or separately, and not everyone gets them all.

Looking back, people sometimes feel that there was a triggering event—infection, injury, surgery, childbirth, or a stressful situation. It is not known whether these types of events are connected with the onset of RA or are coincidental, but there is a widely held theory that chronic infection may be a factor.

RA can wax and wane, or temporarily disappear altogether. A remission can last days, weeks, or longer. A worsening of inflammation, called a **flare**, is connected by some to stressful situations (but not by others, a theme you may have begun to recognize). In a small percentage of cases, the disease progresses in spite of treatment, but new treatments are available. About 10 percent of RA patients will have a complete remission in the first year of the disease, a fact I hung on to with some desperation. Remission or control of symptoms is more often the result of a careful treatment plan.

What's happening in this joint?

In each major kind of arthritis, a different part of the joint is involved. In RA, the joint capsule or **synovial sac** is involved. This capsule is lined with a thin, delicate membrane, the **synovium**, which is one to two cells thick. Clear viscous fluid with the consistency of raw egg white fills the sac. The fluid lubricates the joints and nourishes the cartilage—the smooth, tough, elastic material at the ends of bones that allows them to slide.

The body's defense system normally enters the joints by way of the synovium. Infection-fighting cells release proteins called **cytokines** to create protective inflammation as part of the healing process. In RA, the immune response is perpetuated, and the synovial sac becomes clogged with immune cells and compounds that fuel inflammation. The joint becomes engorged with new blood vessels and begins to grow, a condition called **synovitus**.

What's the worst thing that can happen?

At worst, you'd either ignore the situation or leave it up to someone else—neither of which is happening, because you are reading this book.

You need to know that most people have a controllable form of RA that never moves beyond pain and swelling in the joints. Managing the disease offers a good chance that you will never be faced with the physiological changes that occur in the later, more severe forms of the disease.

Be aware, though, that in time active RA can result in the breakdown of cartilage and bone as well as damage to ligaments, tendons, and joint capsules. X-rays (my X-rays, not yours) show a narrowing of the joint space from the loss of cartilage and erosion of bone on the edges of the joints. Over time, fingers and toes can become misshapen. Small bones in the feet become dislocated, causing pain in walking. Range of motion can become permanently restricted.

It is important to appreciate that rheumatoid arthritis is a systemic disease and not just a joint problem. If it advances, it can also eventually affect other parts of the body—the eyes, heart, and lungs, as well as the membranes that surround these organs. Even though these problems occur only with the most aggressive forms of the disease, it is wise to keep up with routine physicals.

Taking our lumps

Some people, often those with more severe RA, develop small lumps beneath the skin called **rheumatoid nodules**—about a quarter to half an inch across. They develop from the inflammation of a small blood vessel and tend to come and go during the course of the illness. Aside from aesthetics, they do not cause problems.

In a small percentage of those with RA, the glands that produce moisture are affected, a condition called **Sjögren's syndrome**. The resulting dryness in the eyes, nose, mouth, and vagina needs to be lubricated—eyes to prevent damage to the corneas, the mouth to prevent **dental caries**. (Read more about Sjogren's in Month 9.)

And now what?

The prognosis for those diagnosed now with RA is generally good, but it depends a lot on our choices. "Mishaps," wrote James Russell Lowell, "are like knives that either serve us or cut us as we grasp them by the blade or the handle." You can respond to the diagnosis of what is usually a lifelong disease with despair, or you can undertake a well-managed program and lead an active life.

Treatment includes an exercise program, joint protection, weight control, relaxation techniques, heat, and medication. A combination of therapies appears to be the most helpful. Prospects are improved dramatically if you start the program early and aggressively.

What does the future hold?

Powerful new research tools can peer into our cells and even into the molecules in those cells. A nationwide project with the goal of discovering all the genes that contribute to RA has already identified some **genetic markers**. Not all people with RA have these genes, but for those who do, modifying the messages of the genes has become a possibility.

Other research is focused on the multiple steps in the immune system that lead to RA, searching for ways to intervene. Revelations about the functioning of the immune system have made possible a new category of drug, the biologics—expensive, but available now.

Evidence has been gathered to support the idea that there are contributing factors, such as smoking, as well.

Now that we are learning to read the secret language of our cells, changes are coming fast, and you and I are on that wave into the future.

arthritis

_____

arthritis

The logo, above, from the pamphlet I was given when I was diagnosed—reflecting a possible outcome at that time. Below, my reality, more than ten years later.

IN A SENTENCE:

Rheumatoid arthritis is a systemic disease that can now be managed with approaches that address the whole body.

How We Think about RA and Why It Matters

I don't want to be a passenger in my own life.
—DIANE ACKERMAN

Emotions can play a part

When you are diagnosed with RA, your feelings can run the gamut—confusion, fear, anger, grief. You didn't create the disease, and you can't will it away, but how you manage those feelings can affect the course it takes.

I am not a mental health professional, and I don't offer therapeutic advice—or any advice at all, for that matter. I am just a voice from the other end of the boat that we are both in.

What I have learned is that science is solid on this point: fundamental mechanisms of our biology are affected by social and psychological factors.

That idea was once scientific heresy, when the nervous system and the immune system were thought to function independently of one another. As it turns out, the relationship between emotion and health is intimate. Fear and hope are not just feelings. They are physiological states. The brain, as the source of those states, is a gateway to other tissues and organs, including the immune system. The phrase *mind-body connection* carries this dichotomous history; it is as though we had to be reminded of the hand-wrist connection. **Psychoneuroimmunology** is now the branch of medicine that studies the relationships of the mind (psycho), the nervous system (neuro), and the immune system (immunology).

Ninety years ago, Walter Cannon, a psychologist at Harvard, developed a theory known as the fight or flight syndrome. He described the action of the sympathetic branch of the autonomic nervous system as it prepared the body for emergency action. Energy is diverted from internal organs to the muscles. The **hypothalamus**, in response to a warning, secretes a chemical that stimulates the pituitary gland, which in turn makes a molecule that travels to the adrenal gland, stimulating the release of cortisol and adrenaline, raising blood sugar and blood pressure. Ancient ancestors used this reflex when they escaped wolves and hunted mammoths to survive and pass on that trait.

Today, the mammoths hover in museums, and the closest we get to wolves is the donation envelope for their protection. We are living in a physical anachronism, flying into space with primitive bodies. The stress mechanism still serves us well when we are crossing the street when an SUV runs a red light, but such sudden, life-threatening dangers are rare in our lives. We more often experience the chronic stress of stalking projects and lurking deadlines. The body, though, still sees mastodons and wolves. It prepares us to tear across the savannah of the office lobby and down the canyon of West 17th Street, leaping cabs and buses, all the way to our safe treetop lofts.

We know now that stress affects us down to the DNA. Stress unleashes a cascade of chemicals and steroid hormones through these pathways, some of which are inflammatory. Years of chronic stress can wear the body down. In fact, psychological stress is linked to biological age. The direct influence of the stress response on autoimmune disease is not clearly understood, but the indirect impact is so widely acknowledged that stress management is considered to be central to management of RA.

Stress as a factor

The word *stress* was used in the fourteenth century to mean adversity. Engineering adapted the term to describe the load a physical structure bears—at times to the breaking point. Modern psychology defines stress as a condition resulting from the demands of a situation overwhelming a person's ability to cope.

Psychological theories of stress consider the interaction of external and internal factors. Within the same company layoff, there are those who spin into depression and those who pick themselves up and move on. The same external event is modulated by internal factors like coping skills, family support, or beliefs about oneself or the world. The external event may be unchangeable, but coping strategies can be learned.

Short-term stress can motivate change; it can get you moving when you have to. Clearly, it was a good idea to get out of the way of that errant SUV. But the effects of chronic stress are insidious. You may find yourself out of character: reading novels in the wee hours of the night or sinking like a stone past the morning alarm; having no appetite or craving Häagen-Dazs; being low on both temper and memory and high in blood pressure. It can make you sick. Stress will amplify arthritis symptoms such as pain, stiffness, and fatigue.

Processing the diagnosis

The stages of accepting a diagnosis for RA are different for everyone. Some of us are dumbfounded by the news, either numb or sure that it is a mistake. Absorbing the information is a process. Many of us move through a parade of emotions—fear, anger, guilt, and even depression—before we acknowledge this new stage of our lives.

In disbelief, some ignore the diagnosis or go from doctor to doctor: Their thoughts—*I'm not old, I don't deserve this*—are true but not germane. Others pay, both in money and lost therapeutic time, for sham cures.

RA is difficult to diagnose, so if you believe you may have been misdiagnosed, get a second opinion from another rheumatologist. Then choose one to establish a relationship.

When I was diagnosed, I went to a therapist and declared, "I just can't have this diagnosis." I had young sons, a husband, and work, all of which I loved. Years later, barely walking, I encountered the therapist, who was obviously saddened to see my decline. I realized how much easier it was for me to deal with the full-blown disease than it had been to live with the anxiety of uncertainty.

Fear is a normal emotion when you are facing an unknown. Few of us start with any more than a stereotypical idea of RA, one with a bleak future. Fears grow with little understanding of the disease or, worse, old literature: I will lose my job and become a burden, no one will understand, I'll have a life of pain, I will become deformed. The list goes on, but it is not grounded in reality. Some fears are fears of real changes in lifestyle and relationships, but they are not necessarily negative. The **amygdala**, an almond-shaped structure in the brain, integrates the stimuli that evoke fear, but does not sort them by rationality. The result is the chemical stress response. It can be relieved by learning what's true about this disease.

Anger

The only arthritis joke I know is: "Why did the guy with RA cross the road?" Answer: "To kick the chicken."

Frustration with this diagnosis can be expressed in misdirected anger demonstrated in unproductive ways. Some passively do nothing or withdraw affection. Others actively blow up or become sarcastic and hurtful. Either way, it usually makes the situation worse and alienates people when we need support. For many, anger is a passing stage, an expression of an unexamined sense of injustice at the threat of being robbed of health, control, independence, identity, dreams—anger that melts away with the threat and the stress response it evokes.

Guilt comes from the assumption that we are somehow responsible for our diagnosis. Our culture harbors a lingering superstition that we somehow bring illness on ourselves. Perhaps it is egocentric to ask, *Why me?* and assume that the answer has to be of our own creation. Since we are discussing the emotional links to disease, it needs to be stated again here that our thoughts, speech, or actions are not among the causes of RA. We are not responsible. (Month 8 discusses causes.)

Relief can be the feeling for some, those who have been on a quest for a diagnosis and are relieved when they finally get one; the mystery is solved, and they are glad to have a definition.

For most of us, the emotions are more complex, and it takes time to work through them. Feelings can evolve for some like Dr. Elisabeth Kübler-Ross's stages of grieving—denial, anger, depression, acceptance. For others, it is as though they are wandering around in a house of grief, one day in a room of rage, another in a room of frustration, and another in a room of despair.

These emotions are neither negative nor permanent events. They are important signals telling us that something needs attention. We can choose what to do with them. As long as they are out in the light, communicated and examined, they belong to us, and we are not their minions.

It's the buried, denied, festering feelings that putrefy and become a part of the problem. Unexpressed emotion increases the level of stress hormones in the body. Pain is amplified, and a downward spiral of intensified symptoms begins.

It is important to take the time necessary to examine these feelings. It can be like a board game—starting at Go and making the rounds of familiar emotional stops, then going around again. A lot of it can be expensive real estate, depending on how you play the game.

Causes of stress in RA

The symptoms of RA can create stress. Pain contracts our muscles and our psyches. Invisible and intermittent, it can turn stoics into martyrs. No one else can guess what is happening, and we have a tendency to withdraw. We are the least inclined to do the thing that will help the most—move that body. Pain amplifies the sense of hopelessness, a state in which our bodies emit fewer endorphins and pain-blocking chemicals, so the more pain we feel. Pain and stress are the Katzenjammer Kids, one urging on the other.

Fatigue in RA is caused by stress and by the body's reaction to substances released into the bloodstream by activated immune cells. Exercise can be the last consideration, and muscles can begin to atrophy. Eventually, the heart, which is a muscle, can become less efficient. When its ability to pump nutrients and oxygen decreases, muscles tire more easily, increasing fatigue.

Living with uncertainty can be stressful—until you learn to ride the ups and downs of RA. The disease waxes and wanes, sometimes unpredictably, making it difficult to plan. One day is normal, another one is difficult. It's hard to book the calendar if you don't know how you will feel, and it can be awkward to cancel at the last minute.

This book is about how to navigate the best path through these realities in order to live well. And you *can* live well.

IN A SENTENCE:

> *Understanding the emotional component of RA is a key to managing the disease.*

learning

The Role of Stress

> *What lies behind us and what lies before us are*
> *tiny matters compared to what lies within us.*
> —OLIVER WENDELL HOLMES

Styles of dealing with stress

I have a glass on my bathroom sink with a line around the middle marked "half empty" and "half full." The way we respond to stressors can be divided with this old cliché—same glass, different ways of looking at it. Psychology recognizes several characteristics that are common to each point of view.

Those with the half-empty view tend to see things through a negative, pessimistic filter. They tend to generalize the consequences of events (*This will be bad for a long time*), maximize their impact (*It will ruin my life*), and minimize their ability to cope with it (*Nothing I can do will change the outcome*).

Their perception of the enormity of adversity makes them feel helpless and willing to give up, to relinquish control to others, to turn things over to fate. They tend to blame themselves and feel guilty.

Those with the half-full view tend to see things through a positive, optimistic filter. They see themselves as valuable and deserving, and see their defeats as temporary (*This will be a challenge*) and limited (*It can get better*). They tend to separate things beyond their control from things they can control (*I have RA, and there are things I can do to control it*). They don't blame themselves.

Those with a negative outlook can be defeated by emotion, as reflected in our very language: *eaten away by envy* and *consumed by jealousy*. They can become depressed, causing **stress hormones** to flow into the bloodstream and increase pain.

Laughter and a hopeful frame of mind are known to reduce stress. A group of actors performing in a program comprising two plays, one dark and the other a comedy, were found to have altered blood chemistry over the course of the evening.

It has been shown that a person's outlook can affect his resilience, measured by levels and duration of stress chemicals. Most of us move on a spectrum of attitude, seething over Uncle Zeke's brashness but putting up with Aunt Minnie's gossip. Some glasses look fuller than others, and we think little about our choice in the matter.

It doesn't have to be this way

It is true that genetics influences how we look at that half glass, but we are not prisoners of our DNA. Our brains are not set in their structure by the genes that we inherit; they are continuously sculpted by our experience. This revelation earned a Nobel Prize for Dr. Eric Kandel of Columbia University, who demonstrated that our biology is dynamic. We can change. We are changing all the time.

We can *feel* a physical lift from emotion—on wings, on a cloud. Then there is that sinking feeling, feeling low, down and out, bottoming out. Two components, cognition and feeling, are not separate in the brain. Emotion can influence thought, thought can influence emotion. We know that we can choose thought. It does not seem possible that we can thereby choose emotion, but it is true. And it is a useful skill, given that some emotions have such a negative effect on the disease we want to manage.

This is not to suggest that by willpower you can control your condition, or that if you think right you will be cured. Nor does it mean that you are better off ignoring negative emotion.

Simply put, you can manage your health better with a relaxed and positive mind. Having one is a learned skill, one that is further explored in the Learning section that follows. A change in mindset can alter neurochemistry.

How the placebo effect informs your plans

The results of the first **placebo** studies in the 1950s were surprising. Of the people in control groups given fake pills, thought to be inert, a third or more got better. Since then, what was believed to be an imaginary lessening of symptoms has been shown to be a measurable change in brain chemistry.

Dr. Herbert Benson of the Mind-Body Institute at Harvard has found that the placebo effect is influenced not only by the positive belief and expectation of the patient but by that of the health care provider as well. In addition, Dr. Benson cites added benefit if patient and health care provider have a good rapport.

The British physiologist Patrick Wall observed different kinds of placebos, finding that "capsules containing colored beads are more effective than colored tablets, which are superior to white tablets with corners, which are better than round white tablets. Beyond this intramuscular saline injections are superior to any tablet but inferior to intravenous injections. Tablets taken from a bottle labeled with a well-known brand name are superior to the same tablets taken from a bottle with a typed label. My favorite is a doctor who always handled placebo tablets with forceps, assuring the patient that they were too powerful to be touched by hand."

He would like to replace the word *placebo*, which comes from the opening phrase of the Latin vespers for the dead, "I shall please"—an ironic reference to difficult patients who had to be placated with sugar pills. He would like to call it "remembered wellness."

How pain works

Pain signals are carried by nerves in the tissues to the receiving area of the spinal cord, where they are relayed along several points to the brain. Within the spinal cord are cells that can turn pain signals on or off. The "on" cells are important to the reflex that closes your eye before you even see the gnat. The "off" cells interrupt the pain signals. For our survival, the "on" cells are dominant.

Opiates like morphine act by shutting down the "on" cells. But the body produces natural chemicals, like **endorphins**, that mimic the effects of opiates. These natural pain blockers are known to be released in the presence of hopeful emotional states—a conclusion that has been substantiated by several research groups, according to Dr. Jerome Groopman of Harvard.

Putting the stress response to rest

Considerable evidence has been gathered to connect various kinds of soothing emotional experience with benefits to health. A deep sense of calm called the **relaxation response** helps relieve the effects of stress. In a state of mental calm, blood pressure drops, heart and breathing rate slow, and muscles become less tense. When the body is deeply relaxed, it produces more nitric oxide, which is thought to act as an antidote to cortisol and other potentially toxic stress hormones.

Yoga, prayer, meditation, tai chi, or simple deep-breathing exercises are all practices that bring about the relaxation response. Progressive muscle relaxation is another, where muscle groups from the face to the feet are loosened. Some people find a similar effect in repetitive activities like walking, jogging, playing a musical instrument, knitting, or gardening.

Stress can build up over the day. You can plan several breaks to let go of the stress—even if it is only to close your eyes and take a few deep breaths, which can alter your psychological state.

Studies have found that a positive outlook in people with a spiritual life is helpful in adjusting to chronic disease. Spirituality, in this case, need not be organized religion, but a source of hope and solace.

The Luddite solution

Consider the benefits of slowing down. It's just as well to adjust your thinking to the same slow time scale of the disease, since you'll need to develop some patience for its management. Adjusting to treatment programs that may take months to get results is a difficult psychological task in an instant culture.

Our lives have sped up with technology, and many of us are tied to electronics all of our waking hours. What would it be like to turn off La Cucaracha on the cell phone, jingles on the television, ding-a-lings on e-mail, and the beeper on the fax? How about the buzz of coffee and the drone of news?

Wouldn't you rather have a nap? Heresy; no one naps. Even in my kids' preschool, the nappers were of low caste, below the kids wired for action. It takes some courage in a go-go culture to lie down in the middle of the day; we do better at it when we think of it as a job. Fatigue is helped with rest, and so is stress. And a relaxed mind will get you off the good-news/bad-news see-saw to assimilate what you are learning about this diagnosis. If you set the alarm clock, do it to remind yourself that it is time to start your small daily vacation.

What's in it for you, this slowing down, is your chance to arrive in the present moment. It is not mystical hoo-ha but simply stopping and being aware. It has nothing to do with resignation. Mindfulness is a state of paying attention without judgment. Attention is the door to action, and mindfulness brings you to attention. It comes down to this: the future and the past do not hold your answers. Only here and now in a quiet mind can you own this diagnosis and decide how to live with it well.

IN A SENTENCE:

> *Stress has physiologic effects on RA that you can learn to alleviate.*

Making the Necessary Changes to Your Life

Change alone is eternal, perpetual, immortal.
—ARTHUR SCHOPENHAUER

SOME CHANGE is a welcome guest; other change comes uninvited and sets up residence in your life. RA can move in until you imagine it has taken over your very self—your independent, engaged, energetic self. At first you may not realize that you can do a lot to direct the course of that change.

It is said that the best way to live a long life is to have a chronic disease, because then you will take care of your health. It will take time for you to come to that conclusion. I think of the process as a maze that, like a clever computer game, is created by the thoughts of the traveler. On the way to acceptance, there are many dead-end corridors into denial, blame, and anger. This may begin to sound like a morality story; truth be told, it is a kind of cautionary tale. You can get lost in there. I learned some shortcuts, though, and I can show them to you.

Acceptance means redefining yourself—acknowledging matter-of-factly that you have RA. It also means realizing that RA does not necessarily have you. Unless the situation changes (for a few, RA simply disappears), you need to change yourself to manage the situation.

Accepting change is not easy. Accepting change is so difficult that there is a long historical record of peoples that have perished because they held on to entrenched habits despite the needs at hand. For example, the Norse settlement in Greenland did not survive its traditions, which included insistence on a diet based on domesticated animals over culturally unacceptable but abundant seal meat. We are not about to die for the love of a steak (arguably), but we do identify so closely with cultural images that it is hard to let go of them, even when they do not serve our changing circumstances—like supermom and double-overtime guy.

Staying with the anguish of the status quo is one choice. There is something to be said for the payoffs from suffering—martyrdom, pity, attention, victimhood. Not that attractive, but they do have takers.

Preparing for change

In packing for a diving trip, my husband was advised to put half of everything he absolutely needs on the bed and half on the floor, and then to pack the things on the bed. You, at this departure, go through a less arbitrary process of determining what you need and what will be a drag on your progress.

No doubt you have adjusted to new circumstances many times before. RA, though, may require profound change. How do you sort out what to leave behind on the floor? First, you commit to getting well. That may seem like a given, but you may have a steamer trunk full of musts, shoulds, and unexamined beliefs that will weigh down your progress toward wellness.

We have all learned ways of thinking from people for whom the world was a very different place. Since my own mother was born, average life expectancy has risen by almost thirty years. Aging and sickness were believed to be inevitably linked. That is an example of the kind of idea we can leave behind.

Nancy's story

The children's writer Nancy Etchemendy was diagnosed with RA twenty years ago. Her medical options were limited then, and she was in constant pain. She thought she was doing everything she reasonably could to get better, taking her medications and keeping appointments. The doctor had asked her to cut down on the stress in her life, but she had a demanding graphics business, a young child, and a house being remodeled around her—stressors she felt she could not control.

One day, as she painfully walked to her mailbox, a new neighbor introduced herself. The energetic, friendly woman said she lived alone, worked from home, and loved to grow flowers. Nancy told her that she too loved gardening, but she could not do it anymore because of her arthritis. To her surprise, the woman explained that RA used to prevent her, too, from working in the garden and doing much else that she loved in her life. She'd made up her mind, she said, that "there was nothing more important than getting well. Then I just did what it took."

What it took was both fascinating and terrifying for Nancy to hear. The woman quit a stressful job, became a vegetarian, exercised every day, and relocated to an area with better medical care—leaving a husband who refused the move. The point is not that these are the things that are necessary to do, but that this woman committed to getting well and did what it took for her.

Nancy said, "I realized that I only wanted to get well if it wasn't too much trouble for me—if I didn't have to cut back on my work hours, didn't have to let someone help me with my child, didn't have to stop eating steak, didn't have to give up my remodeling project, didn't have to figure out why I was angry all the time. Wanting to get well means wanting it without reservation."

She gave up her business for a more flexible schedule as a writer. She has since become an acclaimed author of children's literature. "In any situation, there is always more than one way to proceed," she says. "Chances are you have more control over your situation than you think, even though sometimes none of your options will seem particularly appealing. Ultimately, you and only you control which way you'll go among the possibilities. This applies to everything from personal decisions to types of treatment and who supplies them."

Starting with a new outlook

Wanting to get well without reservation means a willingness to pay the price, wanting it enough to do whatever it requires. What you give is not only money; you relinquish anything that is in the way of doing what you need to do.

First, take control of your program. It can take a seismic shift to think of your doctor as being in your employ. We have always gone to the doctor to get well, to get the medicine that will make us better. Medical expertise is your invaluable guide, but the decisions are yours. It would be a relief to turn over responsibility, because it is a big job to manage your health. A consultation with your doctor takes a fraction of one percent of your time; it is not possible for the doctor to manage, moment by moment, the rest of your life, and he or she would not presume to do it.

This subject is an ongoing thread in an online RA chat room, to which Carol contributed, "What I hear you saying is, 'take responsibility for your own illness.' I think that is often a hard lesson to learn. But there isn't a magic pill or wizard doctor that can make things instantly better. We have to own our part in our health, whether it is eating right, taking the right meds, and basically everything else."

That "everything else" can involve significant changes, and the question to ask yourself is how far you are willing to go. It may mean changing jobs or location. It may mean confronting yourself honestly and exposing hard truths in a support group or counselor's office.

I just spoke with a young woman who said she wanted to improve her autoimmune condition by exercising. She wanted to swim, but the water in the local pool was too cold. An indoor pool was warm enough but too expensive; her parents would pay for it, but she didn't want to ask them, and anyway it was twenty minutes away, which she said was too far. There was no Plan B, which could have been one of numerous classes, from aikido to yoga, at the community college where she is a student. She had one answer, even though it was no answer.

It took this encounter for me to realize, that's me. My morning exercise schedule at home had stopped because of a shoulder problem that prevented me from using a rowing machine. I had delayed choosing from among other options like biking or trying the health club where my family goes. My reasons—weather, time—had never been measured against my need. It can take the mirror of another person for you to see yourself.

IN A SENTENCE:

> *Committing to doing what it takes to get better is the first step in managing RA.*

learning

Making a Plan

> *Distance doesn't matter; it's only the first step that
> is difficult.*
> — MARIE DE VICHY-CHAMROND

Begin early

Most people with RA can thrive. In spite of the fact that RA
can't be cured, we are walking, biking, and dancing away from
an outdated prognosis of disability and are not looking back.

Treatment used to begin gradually. Joint damage in RA can
begin much earlier than previously suspected, earlier than can
be detected on an X-ray. Now the preference is for early, aggressive treatment as the best way to prevent damage—ideally within
one year after the onset of the disease.

The goal of RA therapy is to restore painless freedom of
movement and prevent damage to your joints. Pain needs to be
controlled, and not only because it hurts. It affects all aspects of
life—mood, concentration, sleep, relationships, eating habits,
and motivation to promote health. Pain can set off an increasingly worsening downward cycle of events. Negativity caused by
pain in turn magnifies the perception of pain, which intensifies
the emotion, and so on. A discouraged person becomes less

inclined to get out, joints become stiffer, and more pain results, leading to depression, muscle atrophy, and widening health problems.

The course is not inevitable

If you take an active role in the control of your condition, you can reverse the cycle. To a large extent, you can take your quality of life into your own hands. The key is knowing how to set goals. It is not just a matter of luck.

Many patients rely on medication alone to ease pain, coping as best they can. Effective management of RA requires more: a sensible combination of routines for exercise, nutrition, work, medication, checkups, and practices that help maintain emotional stability.

Improvement is a slow, methodical process. I hope that I have saved you a lot of time and grief by trying a good number of the harebrained schemes that promise a quick cure. The first ingredient for managing this disease is patience, and the first step is to slow down to the pace of nature. Keep in mind that yanking on a tulip doesn't make it grow. You have embarked on a process comprising many small steps; it will take time for you to feel the effects.

You will need a team

Even for those who already have some pieces of a plan in place, there can be a lot to organize. You can't do it all alone; RA requires a team for consultation and support. The key professional team member is your rheumatologist, a medical specialist who knows the most about RA and who keeps up with rapidly changing information. You will need also to see your primary care physician. You can expand your team as you wish, beginning with your closest family and friends. Other team members may include a physical therapist, counselor, self-help group, and teachers or practitioners of other therapies. As I stood at a drugstore counter asking questions about a medication, I realized that my pharmacist was a member of my team.

However small the team, coordinating the team requires a manager. You didn't sign up for a management job, but you're the one with the inside information, the best person for the task. Think of it this way: it's work only for as long as it takes for the changes to become a way of life. Speaking for myself, it's the life I always wanted but was always too busy to effect—until I had to do it.

Managing your RA team, like any management job, means communicating clearly and keeping track of progress from day to day. You can't do it all at once; you need a plan. It may seem ironic to talk about making a plan when sometimes you just don't feel like planning, but having a plan in place can carry you through those times when you don't feel up to anything at all.

If this is "déjà vu all over again," you may be among the many who set goals only to see them repeatedly dissolve in frustration. Every year around mid-February, a Chicago advice columnist received bags of letters about failed New Year's resolutions. She, too, had gotten nowhere with her intention to become a runner. She reread the stack of resolutions—to lose weight, to quit smoking, to get a promotion—and realized that they were ends with no means to achieve them. She reworded her own resolution: I will put on my running shoes and sweats first thing every morning and go out the back door. That was it. Some days she ran a little, others a little more. As long as she showed up on the porch, she kept her self-respect, which boosted her motivation. Becoming a runner took care of itself.

Creating goals requires a process

Your first act is to get a notebook—one big enough to hold your records and small enough to carry to the doctor's office. There will be too much information to carry in your head, so your binder will be essential. When you are ready, write out your plan. The more specific it is, the easier it will be to follow. The details will be undeveloped when you start, but you can make corrections as you go. It's just a matter of easing into it slowly. Very slowly. (See Month 2 for journal pages.)

Start by setting a long-term goal. You may want to use the goal of having freedom of movement and preventing joint damage. Or, you may want to reword it to be more specific to your life—to hike to a waterfall, to dance at a wedding, to go on a fishing trip, to play the piano, to take your watercolors to the park, to plant sunflowers, to play a round of golf, or to do the three-mile Arthritis Foundation Walk.

Then plan an overview, a bird's-eye look at the changes you eventually want to make. As you do plan, keep in mind that this is a road map, not what you need to accomplish by tomorrow. With no map, there is no direction. Once the overview is in place, you can choose small, achievable steps for each of the long-term changes you want to make. For now, outline the big goals:

1. Assemble a team.
2. Learn to exert control over RA symptoms.
3. Improve physical health.
4. Enhance emotional health.

Now choose what to do in each category. It might look like this:

1. Assemble a team.
   a. Make an appointment with a rheumatologist.
   b. Talk to your family about RA.
   c. Join a support group.
   d. Make an appointment with a counselor.
2. Learn how to exert control over RA symptoms.
   a. Follow the time plan and read this book.
   b. Join the Arthritis Foundation; receive monthly magazine.
   c. Visit the library.
   d. Go online to reputable sites.
3. Improve physical health.
   a. Get a baseline checkup.
   b. Create an exercise program.
   c. Create a nutritional program.
   d. Protect joints.
4. Enhance emotional health.
   a. Pace the day; schedule rest to avoid fatigue.
   b. Learn a relaxation practice such as meditation, visualization, or deep breathing.
   c. Keep social contacts.
   d. Simplify life.

Although these larger goals are broken down, they are still chunks too big to work with. You don't read a book at a sitting or create an exercise plan in a wink. Most important, make changes in your plan as you progress so that you don't set yourself up for failure. Keep long-term goals in mind as you work through short-term goals, and remember that this is a gradual process.

Create bite-sized goals

Continue to break each goal down until you have one single action that you know you can do, and make a contract with yourself to do it. For example, if you want to join a support group, you might break it down and commit to one step:

1. Get information about the support group from your rheumatologist or the local Arthritis Foundation.
2. Phone the group leader and confirm the time, place, and directions.
3. Schedule the meeting on your calendar.

You may need to list other steps as well, such as arranging your work schedule, child care, or transportation. Whatever it takes to do the task, list as many steps as you think could possibly get in the way of the outcome, no matter how small.

To create an exercise program, you might list:

1. Make an appointment with a physical therapist or a trainer, or choose an arthritis exercise program.
2. Check with the doctor.

Choose a long-term goal, say, exercising for thirty minutes five times a week.

Break that goal down to a short-term action plan: for example, doing range of motion exercises for a few minutes each morning and walking fifteen minutes twice a week.

It may take experimentation to break down your goal from miles into yards or steps.

To create a nutritional program:

1. Again, write your long-term goal—for example, take the stress of weight off the joints in your legs and feet.
2. Select a dietary change—to substitute skim milk for whole milk, or have fruit for dessert.

You get the idea. Each category is discussed in other chapters of this book, but only you have your finger on the pulse of your day and know how much is possible. Even after you have reduced your plan to small increments, there is no amount you "should" be doing. Listen to the stress messages from your body and scale back if you need to. Step it up only when you are ready.

Celebrate

When you accomplish a change for a day, celebrate. It may seem contrived or even childish, but there are physiological benefits to rewarding yourself. (Look back to the Living section of this chapter.) Consider the obstacles that you have overcome—pain, fatigue, hopelessness, even boredom. If you have done something today to move toward a goal, reward yourself. Don't wait; celebrate each step. Your accomplishment can be something as small as choosing a salad for lunch, buying a wide-handled tool, or taking the stairs instead of the elevator.

Enjoy taking in a movie, reading a new magazine, soaking in a hot bath, visiting a friend, escaping into a novel, going out to dinner, hitting a bucket of golf balls, or taking out your sketch pad. Choose rewards that reinforce your goals.

I feel a little silly about giving myself accolades for walking past the cookie jar, but I get over it when I sink into my friend's hot tub. This is just a hunch on my part, but I suspect that the unconscious understands actions better than words.

Changing our behaviors is like training a child, or a dog, for that matter, neither of which does better when berated. So an off day is no more than that. If nothing else, we can celebrate treating ourselves kindly when we are not on task. Any excuse for a good time. Now let's begin.

What will you do with your wild and precious self?
— MARY OLIVER

IN A SENTENCE:

> *The first step to managing your RA is making a plan.*

Managing Your Plan

Starting fresh

In Picasso lore, it is said that whenever he decided to start a new style of painting, he moved to a new place, got a new house, and found a new woman. For those of us who have no desire to blow town or dump our mates, the notion that change will uproot us is what makes us so resistant to it. We do, though, have a diagnosis that forces us to take a fresh look. In a way, we need to relocate and change relationships by moving to a new outlook and opening communication with those close to us.

Easy enough for you to say, you are thinking; managing RA is like wrangling Jell-O or catching your shadow. When it's here, you don't feel up to managing anything, and then it's gone so you don't have to. Or, this abstract notion of change feels like just too much to take on.

Educating ourselves and others

Learning to manage your condition is a gradual process. The first step is to learn about RA. Education is the best solvent for helplessness. You're starting your education as you read this book. I encourage you to continue to learn from a range of available information—from scientific to personal. Your fears will be transformed into a realistic assessment as you gather facts.

Use the library. Let the librarians know your interest; they know how to ferret out resources and can set aside material for you as well. Be careful to read the newest information, as the prognosis used to be discouraging. You'll find, too, that the library can be a quiet refuge.

Join the Arthritis Foundation online, by phone, or by mail. You will receive their monthly magazine, *Arthritis Today*. Over the years that I have read it, the magazine has evolved, along with the possibilities for RA. The tone is realistic yet hopeful, and it is an easy and informative read, filled with news and tips for living. Their Web site, www.arthritis.org, is free, as are informative e-mail updates.

Watch the newspapers and magazines. The print media had excellent background material on the new warnings on pain medications, for example. Alert your friends and family to watch for articles in the publications that they subscribe to.

Go online to reputable sites listed in the back of this book. You can keep current on clinical studies and read reports from medical centers across the country. The Web is full of scam cures, so caveat emptor—buyer beware.

Connect with others who have RA:

○ through support groups. Locate them through the Arthritis Foundation Web site or by calling your local chapter.
○ online through chat rooms. You can access one at About.com every evening once you are registered, and you can browse through postings at any time. A sample: "I know how depressing and discouraging RA can be but I just wanted to tell the newbies, especially, not to look for miracles. It takes hard work to feel better with many disappointments along the way."

The more you learn about the course of RA and what you can do about it, the more informed your choices will be, and the more you will feel in control of your life.

What you need to do

As you learn, you will begin to have a clearer picture of what steps you need to take to feel better. One member of a support group uses the acronym SELF—sleep, exercise, leisure, and food. It's a good place to start.

Along with sleep are various types of relaxation that range from rest to visualization exercises. These help reduce stress by increasing awareness of muscle tension and providing ways to let it go. They distract from involvement with illness and pain. When you are relaxed, you are much more likely to do other things to control your symptoms.

Relaxation also involves pacing—alternating periods of work with rest. Initially, the rest periods can be quite long, but they can decrease over time. If they are judiciously planned, they can help protect you from physical impairment. It means finding ways to slow down.

Exercise offers perhaps the most benefit of anything you can do for your overall health. Not only will it help reduce joint stiffness and strengthen your heart, but the endorphins it produces lift your mood and make you feel much more like managing your RA.

Leisure and fun may seem like carrots for the work of managing RA, but they are more than that. Reward is an integral part of your program; the sense of well-being it brings is actually related to altered brain chemistry. The **reward circuits** in the brain (running from the **prefrontal cortex** into lower areas including the amygdala and the **hippocampus**) are rich in **dopamine**, a neurotransmitter associated with elevated feeling. The emotion engendered by reward increases your ability to keep up with the hard stuff. Social rewards have added benefits; they distract from the constant presence of illness by getting you out in the world with others. You can see a pattern developing here, with each act contributing to a chain of responses that support your mood to do more.

Food means attention to nutrition, not a special RA diet. True, you'll find a genre of books and Web sites that tout a cure for RA if you don't eat tomatoes, do take primrose oil, or follow some strict regimen—always sworn to be a miracle for someone. It is true that some people have allergies and report that certain foods are problematic, but those problems are by no means universal. Some studies suggest the possibility of a vegetarian diet as helpful, but a chat room full of people with RA said "no way." The greatest influence that diet has on RA is in relation to the stress of weight on the joints. Your best course is to follow the American Heart Association diet or the new FDA food pyramid—balanced fresh foods.

Your plan

It is one thing to commit to getting well with exercise, good nutrition, relaxation techniques, enough sleep, and enjoyable free time; however, unless you already have such a life, it is quite another thing to pull it off.

There are two ways to go about starting—jumping in or taking it a step at a time. Dr. Dean Ornish supports the cold turkey approach, observing that fast results keep people involved. Such sudden change would have to be undertaken in an organized, directed group, such as the one he runs. Those of us who are managing our own programs do better when the large goals are broken down into an agreeable size. For that, we need to make a plan.

"It's hard enough to accomplish something when you have a good plan. Without a firm plan, forget it," says James Prochaska, a psychology professor at the University of Rhode Island who specializes in studying how people alter their behavior. You need a blueprint to start. When you have a plan, you are less likely to be so overwhelmed that you do nothing. It's not so much a matter of willpower as it is of laying out the steps.

Exercise as an example

Plan to do something, however small, in each of these four areas— sleep, exercise, leisure, food. You will find each of these subjects discussed elsewhere in the book, so we will take just one, exercise, as an example.

First, determine what you need to accomplish: You need to exercise to get your joints moving and reduce stress. Choose an eventual goal. In this case it will include three kinds of exercise:

range-of-motion to reduce stiffness
strengthening muscle groups to keep joints stable
endurance to strengthen your heart, give you more stamina, improve
  sleep, and control weight that stresses joints

Aim to do range-of-motion and stretching exercises every day, with strengthening and aerobic exercise several times a week. Walking, biking, and swimming are often chosen by people with RA, as are yoga and tai chi.

Once you have chosen a long-term goal, break it down to what you can accomplish to start. You may not feel as though you are up to exercising at all, but it is possible to do yoga in a chair. It's a good idea to plan a program with a physical therapist; in any event, clear your program with your doctor.

Set reasonable goals

You have committed to getting well. Rather than making that your goal, set your goals as specific acts toward wellness. Instead of waking up in the morning bummed out over not having achieved the goal of getting well, wake up knowing that you are meeting your goal, say, of doing range-of-motion exercises in the shower. Your internal rewards are emotional (you feel good having done it) and physical (your morning stiffness will be decreased). Some people even process their expectation of continued benefit as a reward. Getting well is a goal so large and complex that it is easy to give up in the face of it, so break it down to create incremental small successes.

In a remarkable story of survival, an injured mountain climber was so daunted by the enormity of the trek down that he was ready to give up his life. He dragged himself to safety with a simple trick; instead of trying to descend the entire treacherous mountain, he focused on only twenty-minute goals. He would otherwise have been defeated by his own mind.

You will find more on the process of breaking down goals in Day 4.

Prioritizing

Setting goals involves not only what you will do but what you choose not to do. It may be that the stage of RA that you are in prevents you from doing everything you once could. Take another look at what is important to your well-being. See what can be delegated or left undone. Lower your standards; can the car go unpolished? Learn to compromise perfection; wash-and-wear clothes save ironing. Learn to say no. I have a *New Yorker* cartoon over my telephone desk: a guy on the phone with his open calendar is saying, "No, Tuesday won't work for me. How about never, does never work for you?"

We see ourselves in certain roles that can be hard to relinquish. I always felt it a duty to be actively involved in my sons' schools. It was not easy to give up much of that participation to my work and rest schedule. And so it goes with roles that we see as inseparable from ourselves.

Living with uncertainty

Some days with RA are better than others, and unpredictably so. Living with uncertainty is a learned skill, one not only for you but your family and friends to master. There are some things in your life, like your work, that you want to plan for. You probably notice patterns in your energy already, and when you begin to keep a journal (see Month 2), they will be apparent enough to help you plan your activities and your rest. There can be hard days, and you can plan for them, too. You may want to arrange to have the option of starting work later, of telecommuting, or of working part time.

Accepting help

We are an independent-minded people. As soon as we can talk, we do it ourselves, and once we've learned to tie our shoes, there is no turning back. Help is only for a two-man job. This is one of the cultural beliefs that will not serve us.

To feel sick is not to be lazy or irresponsible—however guilty we feel in the competitive world we live in. Surely we are not to blame. Even so, it was very difficult for me to ask for help from my family and friends. I did everything myself until I could do no more. It was not until I was bedridden and forced to accept help that I realized that it was not an imposition to ask. It meant a lot for those around me to know how to help.

You are not the only one who sometimes feels helpless in the face of RA; your family feels helpless, too, and being able to do something is a relief. Giving is more of a gift to the giver, it turns out. It's a bit of wisdom that can allow you to ask for someone to pick up children, do the shopping, or bring a take-out dinner.

On the other hand, my son did not consider my asking him to vacuum to be much of a gift to him, but it is a responsibility that contributes to the space he lives in, prepares him for a world that doesn't vacuum itself, and gives him some pocket money. He doesn't always get every corner or get the job done as soon as I'd like; I need to be flexible when I ask for help, to accept what's here in place of an abstract perfection.

Managing your help

When you find sources of support and information, you will need to organize them into your life. It means that you will be at the hub, choosing, directing, and balancing the ingredients of your well-being. Those of us who have gone before you have looked over our shoulders for someone else to come along to do the task; we can save you a kink in the neck and say that there is no one for the manager's job but you.

IN A SENTENCE:

Managing your RA requires a plan that includes personal goals as well as the support of others.

learning

Your Support Network

> *I read and walked for miles at night along the beach . . . searching endlessly for someone wonderful who would step out of the darkness and change my life. It never crossed my mind that that person could be me.*
>
> —ANNA QUINDLEN

Managing your support system

Manager! If it's the last job on earth you ever thought you'd have, we are all in the same boat, at the helm and in a gale. It's high time to assemble a crew.

PRIMARY CARE PHYSICIAN

The first member is a regular primary care doctor (MD)—a general practitioner. If you do not have one, this is the time to make an appointment for an exam. Routine medical care is more important for people with RA. Why?

It's true that new opportunities to control the disease are not reflected in the statistics that show an early death rate for RA. It is still vital for us to stay alert to potential health problems.

A group in a study sponsored by the Arthritis Foundation showed that the RA patients tended not to keep up with basic health prevention that required special arrangements. Appointments can be a nuisance that turn into a part-time job, but keep in mind that problems can develop from inflammation, from side effects of medications, or from the underlying disease process itself. Basic preventive maintenance from your general practitioner, then, needs to be at the top of the management plan, and he or she needs to stay closely involved.

RHEUMATOLOGIST

Your first mate and navigator will be your rheumatologist. This is a crucially important choice. Your relationship needs to be based on trust and confidence. You need to have a doctor that you feel is both competent and caring.

This book cannot take the place of medical advice. It is intended to support your relationship with your doctor by helping you become better informed. Educating yourself will allow you to advocate for yourself and partner with your physician in the management of the disease.

Rheumatologists are trained in general internal medicine and continue their training in arthritic disease for an additional two or three years. They pass rigorous exams to become board certified. A rheumatologist treats arthritis every day and keeps up with rapidly evolving information.

Start your choice with practical limitations, your insurance, and your location. It's best to get a reference from someone who is familiar with the field—your primary care doctor or members of a support group. At one such support group meeting, opinions about doctors flew around the room; the members can be passionate and not always in agreement. It is a personal choice.

You can find out if a physician has been disciplined, suspended, fired, or convicted of a crime (from a Web company called HealthGrades), but beyond the comfort of knowing that your doctor does not belong to a street gang, you are looking for excellence. A word-of-mouth recommendation is really the best.

Short of that, the Arthritis Foundation can provide you with a list of names in your area. You can find contact information for your local office at the Web site www.arthritis.org by keying in Programs and then your zip code. Or call 800-568-4045.

When you call the person you have selected, check to see that your health insurance will be accepted, that the doctor is reasonably accessible, and that the staff is both courteous and available to answer questions. It's useful to get the cross street and parking directions.

This will be a key relationship. Even while you are doing well at maintaining the disease, you will need to check in with your rheumatologist routinely for a long time to come. Treatment for RA is highly individual, requiring a doctor who is a careful listener and observer. Information will come from you, too, and it is important that you have a good rapport. Your best results are from a physician willing to work with you, rather than tell you what to do. Some decisions may be complex or difficult, so a relationship based on trust is important. As you will see as you read on, there is much more to visiting the doctor than dealing with medical symptoms. In rheumatology, there is a premium on the art over the science of medicine; you want to leave with a sense of hope. Over the last decade, there has been a dramatic positive change in how clinicians think about RA, and you need someone who embodies that attitude.

Is the doctor:

easy to talk to? Can you confide in him/her?
able to explain clearly, or did information go over your head?
willing to focus on what is unique to you?
compassionate? Did you leave with a feeling that the doctor can help?

When you consider the importance of your relationship with your rheumatologist, don't hesitate to try another if you are not comfortable. You may as well get it right, because this will be a long, close working partnership. Your appointments will be as frequent as every week to as infrequent as just a few times a year, depending on your need.

Doctors do not have the same luxury to pick and choose patients. Responsibility for the relationship goes both ways, and we could ask some of the same questions of ourselves in the reciprocal role of patient.

NURSES

Doctor's appointments are all too brief. Don't overlook a wellspring of valuable information in the doctor's office: the nurse (**RN**, **LPN**, **NP**; **registered nurse**, **licensed practical nurse**, **nurse practitioner**). While your blood pressure is being taken or while you are waiting for the doctor, ask questions of this qualified professional.

FAMILY AND FRIENDS

Those close to you have many of the same questions you do, but the answers are not coming as fast. Some days you may think that they just don't understand, and, in fact, they may not.

Most family members and friends want to help, but they may not know how to ask. They need to learn enough about RA to work with you. They are landlubbers shanghaied onto this voyage, and they may feel very much at sea.

All they may know are common RA stereotypes of people badly deformed or very old and hunched over a cane. So your first task is to lift the burden of fear that comes with these misconceptions. Tell them that today, most people with RA are rarely handicapped or bedridden; they are usually able to maintain full and active lives. Let them know that although many old people have arthritis, it is not an old people's disease; infants, children and young adults get it, too.

In a more generous era of health care, there were programs for the families of those newly diagnosed with RA. Even now, many rheumatologists encourage family members to come to an appointment.

You will need to set aside time to talk to those close to you about the nature of RA. Explain your symptoms. It is confusing for them to see you feeling fine on some days and fatigued on others. Let them know that it is the nature of the disease to come and go, independent of your desire to go to Uncle Walt's birthday celebration. Ask in advance for understanding if you have to change plans.

During your talk, ask everyone how they feel about your asking for help. Be open about what you are experiencing and what your needs are. Expect that any shift in family dynamics may take some time. Make it comfortable to talk because there will be more to say later.

Help will not come without your seeking it. As obvious as your need is to you, no one can divine your thoughts. For gardening or lifting, you can reach out to a neighbor's kids or to organizations set up to lend a hand. In my town, a local church youth group pays for trips by doing odd jobs, but I would not have known that without calling. There is a wealth of resources in service clubs, Scouts, Guides, temple youth groups, and community centers.

It may be hard to ask for help because you feel a sense of imposition. One experience changed my feeling about that. I once took part in a class experiment that required me to travel with a white cane as a blind person. Dropped off on a corner, I was at a loss to get to a bus stop, but a passerby soon had me by the arm and guided me. There was no shortage of people helping me to my destination, one after another. It had never occurred to me that the city streets were full of souls so willing to assist. We pass each other silently out of respect for privacy, but in a moment many are glad to step forward to meet a need.

Conversely, there are people constitutionally unable to help. "In sickness and in health" is, for some, too much to deal with on the down side. Disease can be frightening or off-putting to them in ways that we can't understand. A therapist I once met calls it the Cootie syndrome—the unreasonable fear that adversity is contagious.

You never know who will stay on board with you. When I became very sick with RA, a neighbor who had been a close friend simply withdrew from my life. I was just as surprised when a casual acquaintance showed up at my bedside in good cheer with a stack of books, which she returned to replenish every so often. It's a hard trick, but it is wise to be grateful for those who come along with you and let go of those who can't. RA acts as a winnowing process, and what you have left are genuine friends. As Oprah remarked, "Lots of people want to ride with you in the limo, but what you want is someone who will take the bus with you when the limo breaks down."

Physical and occupational therapists

It is worthwhile to have a physical therapist (PT) set up your exercise program. There are other resources for exercises, such as classes, trainers, and books, but a physical therapist is trained to assess your particular needs. She can gauge the amount of stress to put on your joints and correct an angle in body position that can mean the difference between help and hurt. PTs can help you manage pain by using heat, cold, or water therapy. Some are trained in massage.

An occupational therapist (OTR) can teach you ways to manage every day activities that may have become difficult by using joint protection techniques or devices. There are certified hand therapists (CHT) who have specialized training in caring for elbows, wrists, and hands.

Get a referral from your doctor to see a PT or OT, and check to see what your insurance coverage is. If you go to PT or OT, you will probably need only a few sessions.

Counselor

When I was diagnosed, I had young children, and I had no idea how to manage. It was helpful to talk over my options with a therapist. This may be a time when you, too, will benefit from counseling. It is a time of transition, and it may ease you along your way.

Ask your doctor for a referral, or get a word-of-mouth referral, to a mental health professional. The title *doctor* may refer to a **psychiatrist**, who is also an MD, or to a **psychologist** with a doctoral degree, PhD or EdD. **marriage, family and child counselors** (MFCC) and **marriage and family therapists** (MFT) are often experienced and less expensive. You can also choose a social worker or a support group leader. Each will help you learn strategies for coping with the complexities of chronic illness. If necessary, you could be referred to a psychiatrist for antidepressants.

Clergy

Even if you are not a member of a religion, a pastor, rabbi, minister, or priest can offer guidance. Many are trained in counseling or can give referrals to other services. You can find a church, synagogue, mosque, temple, or other places of worship listed in newspapers, phone books, and online. If you have been contemplating finding a like-minded group, this could be a good time to benefit from both the support it can offer and the perspective you can offer others.

RA support group

Contact the Arthritis Foundation to find an RA support group in your area. Key into *Events and Programs* and then *Programs and Services*, where you can enter your zip code. A list of support groups and classes will come up, and you can key into any that interest you to get the location and schedule. I found that groups addressing more general autoimmune diseases are less helpful than those specifically addressing RA, but in either case these people are kindred souls. Such groups can provide a good cry, a good laugh, and a lot of useful information. Two thumbs up; highly recommended.

TEACHERS OR PRACTITIONERS OF OTHER THERAPIES

When you decide upon a class for exercise, yoga, tai chi, or any of a number of other helpful practices, count the teacher as a member of your team. Explain your diagnosis and your symptoms, so that he is aware of your goals and limitations. You will find classmates becoming part of your circle. Count a massage therapist or other practitioner as a team member as well.

To find a medical doctor trained to do acupuncture, call the American Academy of Medical Acupuncture at 800-521-2262. Other acupuncturists are certified or licensed (**CA** or **LAc**). In some states, the use of initials such as O.M.D. (Oriental Medical Doctorate) can only be used in conjunction with acupuncturist credentials. Contact the American Association of Acupuncture and Oriental Medicine at 888-500-7999 or www.aaom.org as well as www.acufinder.com to find an acupuncturist in your area.

PHARMACIST

Make use of the option of having your pharmacist (PharmD) step to the counter to explain a prescription. She can point out possible drug interactions and offer suggestions for avoiding side effects. You can also get information about over-the-counter medications or herbal supplements. In some states, your drugstore can offer blood pressure monitors, immunizations, and screens for bone density or cholesterol. It is wise to stay with one pharmacy. Although you need to rely on yourself to keep a record of your medications, the computer list at the drug store will help the pharmacist assess your records.

DENTIST

Particularly if you have the dry mouth sometimes associated with RA, it is important to keep regular dental hygiene appointments. Your dentist (DDS and DMD) can recommend over-the-counter aids or prescribe fluoride treatments to strengthen your teeth. You can get suggestions for taking care of your teeth if painful hands make brushing and flossing difficult.

Let your dentist know what medications you use before starting dental work.

OPTOMETRIST AND OPHTHALMOLOGIST

An optometrist (OD) can examine your eyes for defects and prescribe glasses. The OD degree is granted after at least two years of college and four years in optometry school. An opthalmologist (MD) is a medical doctor specializing in the eyes and can better address symptoms caused by inflammation or medications. An ophthalmologist can prescribe glasses, perform surgery, and prescribe medications. Some insurance policies draw a fine line when it comes to eye exams and will not cover them, even though the symptoms are related to RA. I use a university optometry school for a yearly exam by a graduate student in ophthalmology, overseen by a professor. Occasionally a few grad students will peer into my eyes to observe the effects of Sjogen's syndrome, but I figure that the education is valuable, and the cost is low.

PODIATRIST

A podiatrist (DPM), foot doctor, can remove corns or calluses that contribute to foot pain, as well as prescribe medication. Podiatrists perform surgery, but the small bones in the feet are fused rather than replaced with synthetic joints. It was a podiatrist who initially suspected RA and sent me for a blood test. Also, a podiatrist removed calluses on my shifted metatarsals and relieved the pain at the ball of my foot.

The buck stops with you

This list makes a broad choice of potential sources. Some you may never use, others you may draw on once or twice, a few you may rely on regularly. Some that are hidden in plain sight, like your pharmacist or the nurses in your doctors' offices, are available to dispense wisdom at no additional charge.

It's ironic that you, a layperson, make the decisions instead of these professionals, who have years of training and experience. Here you are, employing these people as resources. Some literature describes your doctor as your manager, and it would be a relief to hand over this job to such a kind and informed person. Some people do. But no doctor has the time to coordinate all the parts of a treatment plan; his experience and knowledge guides your choices. As manager of your health, the buck stops with you. So, Captain, it is time to set your goals and turn to your crew to help you achieve them.

IN A SENTENCE:

You will need a support team to help you manage your RA.

DAY **5**

Visiting Your Doctor

He is the best physician who is the most ingenious inspirer of hope.
— SAMUEL TAYLOR COLERIDGE

The role of your doctor

You've made an appointment with a rheumatologist and are preparing for your visit. (See Day 4 on how to choose a doctor.) Your best sources of medical guidance will be your general practitioner and your rheumatologist. Your doctor has training, experience, and, most important, has you in front of him or her.

You have hired the doctor as a member of your counsel, as a trusted adviser. You are the person running your life, and the choices are ultimately up to you. It's a good attitude to embrace; you will be less likely to detour into blame or resentment when you don't get an outcome that you anticipate. There is a fine line between taking control of your program yourself and following the informed advice of a physician. Trust enriches the relationship, making you open to the benefits of your doctor's knowledge and experience. The best doctors recognize their role as advisers, with the choices as ours.

The writer Nancy Etchemendy and her mother were diagnosed in the same year with RA. Her mother placed herself in the hands of her doctor with the passive expectation that he would make her well. The result is that she is housebound and depressed. Nancy has proactively managed her illness, collaborating with her doctor, and she leads an active life.

The first step is to resolve to do something about your joint pain, and to begin with a doctor-prescribed treatment plan.

Your relationship with your rheumatologist

My rheumatologist says that he has never had a patient that he could not help. It is an extraordinary statement for a modest man, and I believe it. For a doctor to impart hope, he needs to have it himself. It's fair to ask, "Do you believe that you can help me?"

It goes both ways: Do you think you can help him or her? It is, after all, a partnership. Trust and confidence are the nourishment for the working relationship—your trust in the doctor's competence and caring, his trust that you will report openly and honestly on your symptoms and on how well you follow your program.

You are likely to form a long-term relationship with your rheumatologist. You will do a better job of working together if you are sympatico. (Patients with such relationships have even been shown to do better with placebos.) Complicated decisions will come up, requiring well-oiled communication.

There is more to rheumatology than dispensing medications. Since there is no standard treatment for RA, every program is designed individually, and because there is no cure, the program is continually fine-tuned to ameliorate the symptoms or put them in remission.

Your relationship with your rheumatologist has boundaries. Doctors are not therapists, parents, or chums—although their role has elements of each. But he is not a disembodied encyclopedic medical brain attached to a twenty-four-carat gold heart. What's real is that doctors are in a high-stress profession that deals with increasing layers of bureaucracy in the health care system. They have headaches, divorces, teenagers, and commuter traffic. On the other hand, most also have work to which they are devoted. Your well-being is a professional goal. They have entered rheumatology with their eyes open. They know that they are not dispensing cures. They take satisfaction from seeing your improvement and from preventing decline or damage. They are aware that they are in medical territory that is evolving, and many find that challenge the place to be.

In your role as patient, you need to be regarded as a whole person, not a body with arthritis. You need to feel comfortable discussing your fears, asking naïve questions, and expressing opinions and failures with an emotional safety net.

Communication can fail on either side. Most commonly it comes from: a preconceived opinion (e.g., People with RA should not do weight-bearing exercise); undisclosed information (The prescription was too expensive); or a lapse in listening or in not questioning something that is not understood.

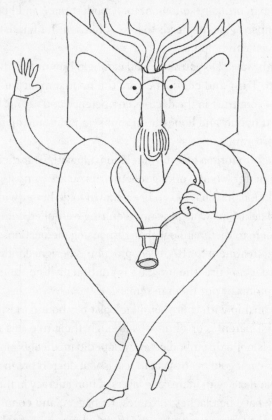

The perfect rheumatologist with a heart of gold and an encyclopedic head.

One rheumatologist was reluctant to tell me that a rash I'd developed was a side effect of the medication he'd prescribed. It took weeks and a dermatologist to establish the link. The rheumatologist felt the rash was less important than my otherwise good response to the medicine, and he did not want to risk my stopping the medication. The omission was made with good intention, but how could I trust him again? If a doctor thinks you do not have choices, Nancy Etchemendy says, you can demonstrate the error of that assumption by choosing another doctor. Both sides need to "tell it true and straight" to develop trust.

Trust is important to your partnership

Trust is a physiological state, according to an ingenious study that allowed researchers to observe in real time how social interactions affect brain activity. Scientists from Baylor University in Texas and from the Californian Institute of Technology used magnetic resonance imaging sensors on players of a cooperative game, fifteen hundred miles apart. As trust developed, they observed increased blood flow in the caudate nucleus, an area of the brain that is also involved in processing rewards. Most remarkably, as days of game playing progressed, the response was stimulated merely by the expectation of trustworthiness before a game even started.

So a dose of the doctor, the healing relationship, could be more than metaphor. (See the description of the reward response in Day 3, Living.) Studies have shown that a patient's trusting rapport with a clinician influences satisfaction, and satisfied patients get better results because they feel that their problems are taken seriously, because they are more motivated to take part in a program, and because they are more open to following professional advice.

Time is restricted for a visit

The most restrictive boundary in your relationship with your doctor is time. You have seen the length of appointments diminish as a result of the requirements of managed care. An appointment may be long enough for a skilled clinician to check your joints and go over your program, but it is rarely as long a time as both you and your doctor would like. With no agenda, communicating your needs can become rushed and confused. Prepare for your visit to make the best use of the time you do have.

Preparing for the visit

A new doctor will need your medical history. If possible, have your primary care doctor forward a copy of your medical records. If you prepare in advance, it will save time for things more important to you. Your records should include:

1. Your family medical history, particularly concerning autoimmune disease.
2. Your medical history.
   a. surgeries, illnesses, injuries to joints
   b. medications or supplements you take, with dosages
3. Lifestyle habits such as exercise or smoking.

The doctor will also need to know your symptoms. It is impossible to remember day-to-day details. Because the pattern and intensity of joint symptoms are the most important clues to a diagnosis, you need to keep notes. You will find more about organizing your journal in Month 2, but for the purpose of your visit to the doctor, you can jot down some information. Pain is so subjective that to say a joint hurts is much less meaningful than a number designation from one to ten. Record:

1. When your symptoms first started.
2. What joints hurt each day.
   a. how much each hurts, on a scale from one to ten
   b. how long morning stiffness lasts and what helps
3. Fatigue level and duration throughout the day.

On your agenda, list your reasons for the visit and what you hope to learn or accomplish. Note your questions as they come to you. Remember, only a few questions will be addressed, so before your appointment, mark the three or four that are the most important.

The examination is hands-on

It may surprise you that your exam begins as soon as your rheumatologist lays eyes on you. A lot is evident to a practiced clinician—swelling, muscle atrophy, favoring a joint—from your posture, the way you move, the way you shake hands.

The examination will be hands-on and should be thorough. You will be asked to move various joints and then passively allow the examiner to move them. The doctor will palpate joints to detect inflammation and tenderness. Individual rheumatologists develop variations in examination techniques. Some have the practice of pressing firmly enough to blanch the examiner's fingernail bed.

Stay focused during the exam, commenting on the joints or allowing the doctor to ask questions as the exam progresses.

You will be asked to make a fist in order to demonstrate the flexibility of your fingers. The joints will be palpated, particularly the first and second joints of the fingers. The wrists will be flexed and rotated to determine range of motion. The elbows will be extended and flexed, both by you and by the doctor.

To examine the movement of your shoulders, you will be asked to touch your outstretched palms over your head and reach back over your shoulder toward the opposite shoulder blade. Your knees will be flexed and palpated as well, and your feet will be squeezed at the base of the toes.

If you have swelling, the doctor will note the consistency in order to eliminate injury as a cause. She will use the back of her hand to feel warmth. The temperature of the knees is normally lower, so a temperature equal to the surrounding skin indicates inflammation. A skilled doctor can feel a difference of five degrees in temperature.

Your heart and lungs will also be monitored in the exam. The doctor will also look at your eyes and mouth for signs of dryness found in a small percentage of those with RA with Sjögren's syndrome (see Month 9 for further information).

Your diagnosis may take time

The medical history, the pattern of symptoms you report, and your physician's examination are the most important guides to your diagnosis. You will probably have lab tests as well. Although they are indicative, there is no test to diagnose rheumatoid arthritis. (Lab tests are described in the Learning section of this chapter.) Symptoms for some types of arthritis develop slowly and may appear similar to other types in early stages, so your doctor may need to watch your symptoms to confirm a diagnosis. The process may take more than one visit, even though she wants to make a diagnosis as soon as possible. Early aggressive treatment gives the best chance of avoiding the erosion that can start in the first one to two years. There is only short-term data, but it strongly suggests that current patients can do well if they follow the new principles of therapy described in this book.

It takes time to find the right drugs

Based on what your doctor has learned, she will suggest a medication. Often, this will be a **DMARD** (disease modifying antirheumatic drug) that can influence the disease (see Days 6 and 7 for explanations of drugs). Be sure you understand what medication is being prescribed—the name, the dosage, how often to take it, whether to take it with food, and when to expect results. It takes time for the drug to become effective, and it may take more than one trial to determine what will help you. It is not a question of the doctor's ability; the efficacy of drugs varies with the individual, so hang in there.

Report all of your symptoms, even if it feels like you are crying wolf. It is important to be aware of, but not obsessive about, potential side effects, including allergies. Question your doctor and also use other resources to learn about your medications. Your research will allow the appointment to be focused on what is unique to you.

Keep your records

Record the date and content of your visit in your notebook. Ask that your rheumatologist share information with your general practitioner, whose address and fax number you will need to bring. The general blood work will not need to be done by both offices.

Bring your calendar to make your next appointment. You will schedule visits to your rheumatologist as frequently as weekly at first to eventually a few times a year. You may want to choose one day in the week for appointments and errands. I like to take the first medical appointment of the day or the first after the lunch break because a doctor is less likely to be behind schedule for those appointments.

Do I have the right doctor?

For me, the simple test of whether the doctor is right for me is this: do I feel a sense of hope when I leave the office? When I was first diagnosed, I went to a lecture on RA given by a rheumatologist at the local hospital. It was an hour of depressing facts, and I wept as I drove home. I chose a doctor for myself with a buoyant spirit who filled me with hope, even when I was in a wheelchair. I saw him yesterday and discovered that, even though I am in remission, the earlier systemic damage to my shoulder may require replacement surgery. Still, I left hopeful and glad for the guidance. I wish such a physician for you.

IN A SENTENCE:

> *Choose a doctor you can communicate well with, and arrive at appointments well prepared to make good use of the time.*

learning

Medical Tests

How the lab tests are helpful

No lab test can accurately diagnose RA. Attempts have been made to correlate data from various tests on an individual to come up with a diagnostic that is better than the sum of its parts, but there are too many variables to derive an accurate indicator. The tests are not useless, however. They can narrow down possibilities, suggest a prognosis, evaluate symptoms, and monitor the side effects of drugs.

After you are diagnosed, you may wonder why you need to have frequent blood tests. Both your primary care doctor and your rheumatologist will want to keep track of your health status. Some drug side effects need to be monitored because they initially show no symptoms, like a decrease in white blood cell count or liver damage.

Request that lab results by the rheumatologist be forwarded to your primary care doctor, and have tests done by your primary care doctor sent to your rheumatologist. That way, both doctors will stay informed, and you won't have to repeat tests, like the routine blood count, that are ordered by each office.

Blood for these tests is taken from a vein in the arm. The following tests are those most often ordered by rheumatologists.

Complete blood count (CBC):

A complete blood count is a routine test given to indicate your general health. It provides information about the proportion of white and red cells in the blood. The information can detect anemia or infection, which can cause symptoms such as fatigue or fever. The CBC is also used to monitor the response to some drugs.

The test usually includes:

1. *White blood cell count.* The white blood cells, or **leukocytes**, are the immune cells. (See Month 7 to learn how they function.) A raised count can show the presence of infection.
2. *Leukocyte types.* The five kinds of leukocytes play different roles in the immune response. The proportion of each type can indicate infection, allergic reaction, or other conditions.
3. *Red blood cell count.* The red blood cells distribute oxygen from the lungs and return waste carbon dioxide to the lungs to be exhaled. A low count can indicate anemia. About five million cells per microliter is average, with the count varying by sex.
4. *Hematocrit (HCT).* This test measures the volume of red blood cells, given in a number indicating the percentage in the total volume of blood. A low hematocrit can be an indicator of RA as well as of anemia.
5. *Hemoglobin (Hgb)* is the oxygen-carrying molecule in red blood cells that gives the blood its red color. The test determines the distribution of oxygen throughout the body.
6. *Red blood cell indices.* The size of red blood cells and concentration of hemoglobin, measured by these tests, can indicate anemia.
7. *Red cell distribution width (RDW).* Determining whether the red blood cells are about the same shape helps classify types of anemia.
8. *Platelet count.* The blood platelets control blood clotting. With too few, bleeding can be uncontrolled; too many can cause atherosclerosis.

Rheumatoid factor (RF)

Rheumatoid factor (RF) is an autoantibody produced by B cells in the joint lining (see Month 7). The antibody, usually the immunoglobulin IgM, can attach itself to normal body tissue, resulting in damage. It is present in most people with RA, but not in all. As a diagnostic tool, the test is considered along with other information.

Rheumatoid factor is used as a prognostic indicator, with high RF an indicator of severity, and RF negative status associated with a better prognosis. The measure can vary in an individual from test to test. When RA is treated successfully, RF titer tends to fall. However, changes in RF titers often lag behind other markers.

The RF test can give both false positive and false negative results. Some healthy people have an elevated level of RF. A positive test can be caused by RA, but it can have other causes as well, such as hepatitis, viral infection, leukemia, mononucleosis, lupus, or multiple vaccinations. The blood pressure drug Methyldopa can increase the amount of RF detected by the test.

The RF test is a better diagnostic for Sjögren's syndrome, an RA-related condition. About 80 percent of patients with this syndrome have high amounts of RF in their blood.

Two different methods of testing for RF, the **agglutination** and **nephelometry** tests, mix the blood sample with antibodies and measure the response.

ERYTHROCYTE SEDIMENTATION RATE (ESR)

The **erythrocyte sedimentation rate** (ESR) or sed rate is the most commonly ordered lab test to assess disease activity. It is not in itself diagnostic, but it determines the severity of inflammation and is used to monitor the progress of RA treatment.

The degree of elevation can suggest disease progression; a sed rate over thirty suggests active inflammation. A high sed rate at the outset does not predict bone erosion, but over a long period of time it does. It can be an indicator when there is no rheumatoid factor, and is said to be a better predictor than **C-reactive protein** (CRP).

The sed rate measures how quickly red blood cells (erythrocytes) settle in a test tube. Certain proteins present in inflammation adhere to red cells, causing them to stick together and fall more quickly to the bottom of the tube. The rate at which they fall in an hour is the ESR.

There are other possible causes of an elevated sed rate beside RA. Other tests are done in conjunction to come to a diagnosis.

C-REACTIVE PROTEIN (CRP):

A CRP test, like the more commonly used sed rate above, is used to monitor inflammation in rheumatoid arthritis and other autoimmune conditions.

It may be a positive indicator for patients with no detectable rheumatoid factor.

C-reactive protein (CRP) is produced by the liver in response to the presence of inflammation in the body. The cause can be an autoimmune response or bacterial infection. The test measures only the amount of CRP, so other tests are necessary to determine the cause.

ANTINUCLEAR ANTIBODY ASSAY (ANA)

The **antinuclear antibody assay** (ANA) test is another measure of autoantibodies. About 5 percent of people have elevated titers, and about half of those have autoimmune disease. The ANA test does not indicate the presence of disease or determine its nature. Once again, it is a test used in combination with an examination, medical history, and other tests.

JOINT FLUID ANALYSIS

If there is an unanswered question as to whether your condition is an infectious type of arthritis or gout, there may be an examination of joint fluid. The fluid, also called synovial fluid, is examined under a microscope for the presence of bacteria, crystals, and inflammatory blood cells.

In a normal joint, a small amount of fluid acts as a lubricant and a cushion. In an inflamed joint, swelling is caused by increased fluid, and that fluid will hold clues to the cause. The fluid sample is usually removed from your knee, but it can also come from another major joint.

Occasionally accumulated fluid can be drained with this procedure to relieve pain. The same procedure may also be used to inject medications, such as corticosteroids, into a joint.

If you are to have a joint fluid analysis, it can be done in your doctor's office by your rheumatologist or a health care professional trained to do the procedure. Talk to the doctor about the need for the test and about any risks. Tell the doctor if you have taken aspirin recently, are taking any blood thinning medication, NSAIDs (see Day 6), or are allergic to any medication, including anesthetics. You may not need to undress, depending on which joint is involved. The procedure should take only about fifteen minutes, and is often done with a local anesthetic injected at the site. You will be asked to sign a consent form.

X-ray

X-ray is not used as a diagnostic tool because it cannot detect early erosion of cartilage and bone. It can help evaluate progression of advanced RA or determine if symptoms come from injury.

The HAQ, another measure of function

Over the last two decades, assessment of RA—as of all health—has undergone a change from reliance on lab tests, such as those listed above, to an emphasis on patient evaluation. The Health Assessment Questionnaire (HAQ), developed in 1980 by Stanford University Arthritis, Rheumatism, and Aging Medical Information System (ARAMIS), was among the first patient reporting tools. It has since been used over two hundred thoursand times to evaluate progress. It is the most commonly used form for assessing physical function in rheumatoid arthritis trials. It is available in more than sixty languages.

Information gathered by the HAQ was a catalyst for a dramatic shift in RA care—the inversion of the therapeutic pyramid. Patients once started treatment at the bottom of the pyramid, with the most benign drugs; now they are started at the top, with the most aggressive therapies as early as possible. No doubt the HAQ will play a role in the evaluation of the improved outcomes of those diagnosed today.

You may be asked to fill out the HAQ. It is a twenty-question index that asks you to report the degree of difficulty that you may have in rising, dressing, eating, walking, taking care of hygiene, reaching, gripping, running errands, and doing chores. There is also a pain scale to be filled out. It is usually self-administered. With scores of 0 to 1 for mild to moderate difficulty, 1 to 2 moderate to severe disability, and 2 to 3 severe to very severe disability, the average for RA patients is 1.2. There are other similar scales, or your physician may have a form for you to copy and fill in for each visit.

IN A SENTENCE:

> There is no diagnostic test for RA, but your doctor uses tests to help define your symptoms, monitor your progress, and ensure the safety of drugs.

Taking Drugs for RA

DRUG TREATMENT is part of the program for most of us with rheumatoid arthritis. It is easy to be cynical about drugs. We have gone through a media blitz that has made some pain medications the hottest selling drugs in the world, only to find out that they create a risk to the heart.

But cynics stew in a toxic brew that is not good for what ails us. We are better served by being skeptics, picking our way through confusing messages to make informed choices. Balancing the risks and benefits of drugs that can help us is done with the advice of a doctor. The information that follows is purely educational, and does not presume to prescribe. The drugs I take work well for some but not everyone. The risks I have chosen to accept for side effects may not be your choices.

Drugs alone do not make an RA program. A drug can make an impact, but more often there is a synergy among all of the additional elements—exercise, good nutrition, relieving weight on your joints, and relaxation techniques.

It is remarkable that the extensive commentary on the Vioxx debacle presents the problem as being what pill to take to replace the withdrawn or risky medications. Rarely is mention made of the proven contributions of exercise and relaxation practices to pain control.

A critical window of opportunity exists early in the disease, the time with the best chance of preventing irreversible joint damage and achieving remission. Disease-modifying therapy is best started within the first months, or as soon as possible. Pain-suppressing drugs, analgesics, and **nonsteroidal anti-inflammatory drugs (NSAIDs)** do not modify the disease.

Your inner skeptic can take one look at the potential side effects of a medication and back away. Terrifying lists cover every bardo of hell. If I were perverse enough to choose a favorite, it would be one cited as rare for a drug that I swallow every week: "sudden death." Faced with what feels like a devil's bargain, you will value the guidance of a physician you trust in finding the safest, most effective drugs.

Some history of arthritis medications

In the seventeenth century, rheumatism was treated with Peruvian bark, which contains the antimalarial agent quinine. Modern medicine uses the antimalarial hydroxychloroquine sulfate, known as Plaquenil, for RA. In the eighteenth century, rheumatism was treated with willow bark, which contains salicylate. In the nineteenth century, the Bayer Company used the willow cure to manufacture acetylsalicylic acid—aspirin. It became the standard for treatment of rheumatic disorders. The invention of the X-ray allowed a kind of helpless observation of the progression of RA.

By 1929, injections of gold salts were used, inexplicably, to relieve arthritic pain. In 1948, two discoveries were made that have influenced RA treatment ever since. Steroid hormones were found to have remarkable anti-inflammatory effects, and the antibody known as the rheumatoid factor was isolated in the blood of people with rheumatoid arthritis. A test for RF was devised. A synthetic cortisone, Prednisone, was introduced in 1955, and it became widely used. The drugs available provided some relief, but for many the relief was not lasting or came with serious side effects. The first drugs to slow or stop the course of RA, the DMARDs, and now the biologics, have changed the prognosis of a once debilitating disease.

Educating yourself about pharmaceuticals

Ask your doctor about any drug proposed for you. Why choose it? What is it expected to do? How long does it take to become effective? What are the possible side effects? Read further about it on a responsible Web site or in other resources. Speak with your pharmacist about it.

Some drugs were adapted for RA from use for other diseases, in the whatever-works school of drug therapy. It is not known how they work, or why they work for some people and not for others. No combination of medications is effective for everyone. Drugs act differently on different people, and it takes patience to find what is right for you.

Know what the available treatment categories are and how they affect the disease process. (See the Learning section of this chapter and the next.) Know how to protect yourself from invisible side effects; some drugs require regular lab tests, eye exams, or hydration. Be aware of any symptoms of allergy to a medication. Some drugs cannot be taken with particular pre-existing conditions or pregnancy. Before taking even an over-the-counter drug, check with your doctor, because medications can act differently in combination; two drugs that irritate the stomach lining, for example, can be more than twice as dangerous as one.

Dealing with side effects

Some side effects disappear as your body adjusts to a drug. Others are alleviated by taking the drug with food, replacing drug-depleted nutrients, or taking other medications to ease the effect. Sometimes cutting the dosage or dividing the medication into smaller, more frequent doses helps. It can be necessary to change to another medication. The balance of benefit with discomfort or danger is a judgment to make with an experienced doctor. Once you decide, the right drug can enhance your life. From an online RA chat room: "It's absolutely amazing what finding the correct medication combo can do."

Over-the-counter drugs

If you consider over-the-counter drugs to be cheaper than prescriptions, look at the big picture. Check the cost per milligram and the inconvenience of more pills to juggle. Most health insurance plans pay only for prescribed medications. If you are using high anti-inflammatory doses of over-the-counter acetametaphins, you need to see a doctor. Most important, you may be losing precious time in delaying the start of disease-modifying drugs.

Taking generic drugs

When a drug patent expires, any company can manufacture it as a generic with approval of the FDA. A patent can be granted at any point during the development of a drug and expires twenty years after the date of filing. FDA testing allows some variation, so the filler or absorption rate may not be exactly the same in a generic.

The difference in cost between generics and brand name drugs is significant. Insurance often gives better coverage for generics. If you have reason to prefer a brand name drug, your doctor has the option of ordering a prescription with no substitution permitted.

Disposing of medications

It may be that you will change medications in the search for the right combination for you. Typically, unfinished prescriptions have been flushed down the toilet, but the Environmental Protection Agency cautions you not to. Sewage treatment facilities are not designed to filter out pharmaceuticals, and septic tanks can introduce toxic waste into the water table. Some pharmacies will dispose of the drugs. You can also take them, along with your spent batteries, as hazardous household waste to your recycling center, although some will not accept controlled substances (for example, morphine, or Tylenol with codeine), which you may have to take to a pharmacy. For further information, see the Resources section of this book.

Taking medications

Report to your doctor any adverse effects from drugs you are taking, even if you feel like Chicken Little. Report signs of infection if you are taking disease-modifying antirheumatic drugs (DMARDs) or the new **biological response modifiers (BRMs)**. Also, check with your doctor before getting vaccinations.

It's not always easy to remember to take medications, especially if they are not taken every day. A quarter of Americans either don't have prescriptions filled or don't take the prescriptions. They are more likely to continue medication for an acute problem than a chronic problem. Those of us with

RA are compelled by our condition to find ways to build the habit of taking medication into our days or weeks.

Putting my medication where I am going to encounter it helps me remember. A container with a compartment for each day of the week is helpful. Some people like to mark a chart on the side of the pill bottle. During one busy week, I could not recall whether or not I had taken my injection, so I now mark the packets with the date they are to be given.

If you find yourself restarting a medication that you have taken before, check the expiration date. If you have stored it in a cool, dry place, it should be fine, but if it has been in the bathroom cabinet steaming during months of hot showers, don't take a chance on its strength. If you are not sure, discuss it with your pharmacist or dispose of it.

Also, if you have difficulty swallowing some pills or are giving them to a child, they can be crushed and placed into gelatin capsules that you can buy from your pharmacy. Some pills can be crushed and mixed with food. In either case, bring it up with your pharmacist.

The showstopper for many of us with RA is child-proof pill bottles. If there are no small children in your house, your request for flip-top caps can go on your record in the pharmacy and come with every order.

If your RA is flaring and there is an important event coming up for you, speak with your doctor about the possibility of rearranging your medications. All of the other pain-reducing strategies can help you enjoy your day also.

IN A SENTENCE:

> *The process of finding the most helpful drugs for your RA will require a systematic approach with your doctor.*

learning

Drugs for Pain

Three categories of drug that do not influence the course of RA are taken for pain:

Analgesics, from the Greek meaning "without a sense of pain," include over-the-counter acetaminophen and prescription opiates.

Nonselective nonsteroidal anti-inflammatory drugs (NSAIDs) are numerous prescription and nonprescription drugs, including aspirin.

Selective NSAIDs, also called cox-2 inhibitors, the newer drugs designed to avoid side effects of nonselective NSAIDs, have been found to have other serious side effects.

If you contemplate taking any of these medications, you and your doctor are the best judges of what is best for you. Don't hesitate to ask questions or to get another opinion, particularly if you have a preexisting condition or anticipate becoming pregnant.

Note that brand names are mentioned here as examples, not recommendations, just as the absence of a brand is not a comment on its efficacy.

Analgesics

Analgesics are drugs that relieve pain without having an effect on the course of the disease. They may be safer for people who cannot take NSAIDs because of allergies or stomach problems. Acetaminophen is one of the most common ingredients in over-the-counter medications such as Anacin, Excedrin, Tylenol, and generics; it is the safest pain reliever currently known, although it is toxic in overdose. Prescription analgesics include the opiates; examples are codeine, morphine, and oxycondone.

Analgesics work by blocking the pain receptors in the brain. They take effect quickly, usually within an hour, and last for up to eight hours. Sometimes acetaminophen is combined with other substances such as caffeine, which can keep you awake, or antihistamines, which can make you lethargic.

It is commonly suggested that you take analgesics for no more than ten days. Check with your doctor about combining acetaminophen with any other drug, especially with blood thinners. If you take more than three alcoholic drinks a day, it is possible to cause liver damage. Because aspirin acts as a minor blood-thinning agent, almost all people who take it have blood loss through the bowel, requiring blood tests for those on high doses.

Topical creams may help. Salicylates block pain through the skin (Aspercreme, Ben-Gay, and Flexall, among others). Others work by distracting nerves with an irritant, which is unpleasant to get in your eyes. Some contain capsaicin, an ingredient in pepper (Zostrix); or eucalyptus, menthol, camphor, or turpentine oil (Icy Hot).

Many nondrug treatments help ease pain, including relaxation techniques, heat and cold, and massage.

Nonselective NSAIDs

Nonsteroidal anti-inflammatory drugs (NSAIDs) are among the most frequently used drugs in the U.S. They include ibuprofen (Advil, Motrin), naproxen (Aleve), and salicylates (aspirin: Anacin, Bayer, Excedrin)—over twenty medications. They come from different chemical families and are not interchangeable. Some are better than others for some individuals.

The major benefit of these drugs is relief of pain, and at a high dose, of inflammation, although they do not alter the course of the disease. The serious side effect for some people is gastrointestinal problems, which cause more than 100,000 hospitalizations and an estimated 16,500 deaths annually, according to the U.S. Department of Health and Human Services. People most likely to suffer serious side effects are those who are older, are taking high doses for long periods, and are also taking steroids.

Pain signals are created in affected tissues by enzymes called cox, short for **cyclooxygenase**. The resulting reaction produces inflammation. Non-selective NSAIDs inhibit the production of two forms of the enzyme, cox-1 and 2, thereby shutting down the pain signals. Because cox-1 was known to help maintain the lining of the stomach, blocking it was considered to be the cause of gastrointestinal problems. The selective NSAIDs were developed to block only cox-2.

All NSAIDs can raise blood pressure and affect kidney function. Medications to reduce stomach acid are often prescribed with NSAIDs; however, a study published in *The Journal of the American Medical Association* shows that these acid blockers may increase the risk of pneumonia. Some rheumatologists now use lower doses of NSAIDs or recommend an analgesic, acetaminophen (Tylenol).

It can help to take an NSAID with food or change the time it is taken. Some people have fewer side effects with one NSAID than with another. Sometimes lowering the dosage or increasing it gradually avoids problems. Other people remain willing to take a cox-2 inhibitor despite the risks described below. In any case, this is a subject to be discussed with a doctor, with consideration of any supplements or other drugs involved.

NSAIDs can cross the protective barrier that prevents toxins from entering the brain, disturbing the functioning of the central nervous system. The result can be changes in mood or sleep patterns, headaches or ringing in the ears. Use of high amounts of alcohol increases the gastrointestinal toxicity of the NASAIDs.

Selective NSAIDs, the cox-2 inhibitors

Nonselective NSAIDs, such as aspirin, ibuprofen, and naproxen, were thought to block an enzyme considered to be protective to the stomach. It came as great news to those with the resulting stomach problems to learn of the availability of the new selective NSAIDs. The theory was that by suppressing only the cox-2 enzyme, pain and inflammation would be relieved while leaving the protective cox-1 in place. Selective NSAIDs are not more powerful as anti-inflammatory agents than the nonselective NSAIDs and do not alter the course of the disease, so relief from a side effect was intended to be their advantage.

There was need for such a drug, and marketing fanfare made the cox-2 inhibitors the most commercially successful drugs to date. Then came the revelation that drugs in that category—first Vioxx and subsequently Celebrex and Bextra—increase the risk of heart attack and stroke. All also have the rare risk of skin reaction.

NSAIDs may interact with other drugs

If you take drugs for other medical problems or over-the-counter drugs for RA, there may be drug interactions with NSAIDs that can cause side effects or decrease effectiveness. Among the drugs that may interact are some antibiotics, anticoagulants, corticosteroids, diuretics, lithium, oral diabetes drugs, and penicillin. Your doctor may need to regulate dosages.

The FDA warning on NSAIDs

The news has been confusing and disturbing. With evidence from studies done on the selective NSAIDs, showing risks to the heart, the FDA has ruled that the risk applies to all of the drugs in the category, with the exception of aspirin. Although the selective NSAIDs were supposed to be safer on the stomach than older pain pills, it has been reported that it had not been proven to be the case with Celebrex and Bextra. None of the three selective NSAIDs has been proven to ease pain better than older pills, and all three pose a risk to the heart.

The FDA has asked for strong warnings to be placed on prescription painkillers, both nonselective NSAIDs (Mobic, Naprosyn, Motrin, Voltaren, and others) and selective NSAIDs. This includes over-the-counter drugs like Advil and Aleve. Few studies have been done on the long-term effects of these drugs, which have been prescribed for the lifetimes of many patients.

Some doctors feel that warning labels on all of the NSAIDs could trivialize the danger of the more toxic drugs. Although these drugs are sometimes listed in order of gastrointestinal toxicity, the added heart risk complicates comparison. There is some evidence in the research that the medications that are the least toxic to the stomach may be the greatest risk to the heart and vice versa. Vioxx was easiest on the stomach and probably the most potentially harmful to the heart. "We don't have enough data to rank-order these risks," concludes Dr. Steven Galson, acting director of the FDA's Center for Drug Evaluation and Research.

At this point, a doctor must consider a patient's history of heart or stomach problems if an NSAID is to be prescribed. Also, as always, one medication may work for one person and not for another—a fact to add to the equation of risk.

The FDA has no authority to require further trials of approved medications. Furthermore, government officials have acknowledged the difficulty of discovering the links between drugs and common health problems that can stem from other causes.

Over-the-counter pain pills are considered safe in low doses of short duration, with some experts concluding that naproxen, the ingredient in Naprosyn and Aleve, is probably the safest among the NSAIDs. Dr. Alastair Wood, chair of the advisory panel to the FDA that studied the selective NSAIDs, suggested that patients start with naproxen, with the addition of an over-the-counter heartburn pill like Prilosec if they develop a stomach reaction.

As of this writing, the selective NSAID Vioxx has been withdrawn from the market and the FDA recommends that Bextra be withdrawn. The advisory panel recommended that another selective NSAID no longer be advertised, but the FDA cannot ban the advertising of an approved drug. Dr. Galson said that banning ads for one drug made little sense when similar pain pills have similar risks.

As a result of these findings, millions of people felt they were faced with a no-win decision. Dr. John Klippel, the medical director of the Arthritis Foundation, urged caution in the use of selective NSAIDs for people at risk of cardiovascular complications. He also remarked that patients should be able to make informed choices for themselves based on disclosure of the risks involved. In a letter to the FDA, his recommendations included: return of Bextra and Vioxx to the market, reconsideration of the warning for all NSAIDs, better monitoring of approved drugs to assess risks, improved consumer education, and increased public participation in evaluation of arthritis drugs. Dr. Klippel reminds us that "Managing arthritis means doing more than taking drugs. Most people don't pay attention to diet or exercise, and both can help relieve arthritis pain."

IN A SENTENCE:

> *Pain medications can be used to relieve discomfort in active RA, but they do not alter the disease.*

living

Frequently Asked Questions about RA

DR. KENNETH SACK, in the foreword to this book, cites four common questions a person asks when newly diagnosed: What caused my disease? What will this illness do to me? Can I be treated safely? Can I still have a life? His answers to me when I asked those questions were those of a great physician—what is known and what is not known, infused with hope.

I wonder at how I left his office with so much confidence, not always under my own power, with answers that were at best uncertain. In fact, the answers to most questions about RA are uncertain. As I research this book, I begin to see that one of the gifts of this disease is that it casts us into an unknown; we have no choice but to find our firm center, lest we be lost in it.

What caused my disease?

There are different degrees of RA, from very mild to the more inflammatory disease that most of us have. We know that there are genes and combinations of genes that predispose us to RA, but the cause isn't so simple. Not all people with the disease have the genes that have been identified so far; some people who have the genes don't have the disease—including one of the researchers on a fascinating national study of RA genetics. (See Month 8.)

No genes act alone. Their influence on the body depends on the actions of other genes and on environmental factors, which, in RA, include smoking and stress. People with certain gene combinations and environmental factors are at higher risk of developing RA, but the demarcations among nature, nurture, and wellness shift, making them at best difficult to know.

What is known is that you did not cause RA by any thought, word, or deed—regardless of any sense of guilt or responsibility you may have.

What will this illness do to me?

Probably nowhere near as much as literature more than a few years old would lead you to believe, and probably far less than it has done to those who have gone before you. I repeat, in hopes you will believe this: Most people who actively participate in the management of their RA can lead an active and satisfying life. There are new drugs and a new way of looking at prescribing, both earlier and in combination. But, again, the program involves more than drugs; exercise, good nutrition, and stress reduction play a part.

Those with more difficult symptoms may have a sudden and overwhelming onset as well as persistent high levels on tests such as the rheumatoid factor and C-reactive protein (explained in Day 5). The answer is not carved in stone; these tests are not considered to be dependable diagnostics.

It is more to the point, to paraphrase John Kennedy, to ask not what this illness will do to you but what you will do for this illness. People with RA are able to manage it as never before, and this book will help you start your program.

Can I be treated safely?

Reading the list of possible side effects for any drug can be like a tour of the netherworld. To weigh these risks, you will need the educated and experienced advice of your doctor. The decision to take a medication will be yours, though, and you will do well to inform yourself of the choices (see Day 6 for a discussion of drugs).

Many medications that have serious side effects with prolonged use, like corticosteroids, are relatively safe when used for a short time. The side effects of pain medications, the NSAIDs, have been in the news, with some pulled from the market and others requiring a warning label. These drugs suppress pain but do not alter the course of the disease. You may want to

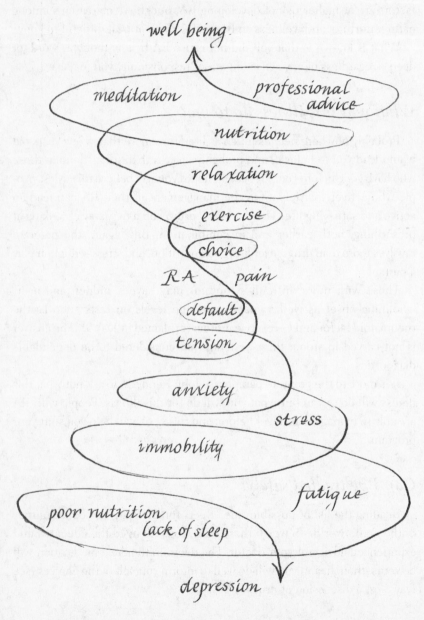

consider pain-reducing alternatives like exercise and relaxation techniques if you want to lessen or eliminate your need for these drugs. (See Day 2 for a discussion of stress and pain, and Month 5 for pain-relieving practices.)

Most people with RA take disease-modifying drugs that are monitored for side effects through regular blood tests. Long-term data is not yet available for the new biologics, but despite some reported susceptibility to infection they are considered to be relatively safe at this point.

Can I still have a life?

Ah, at last a simple answer: Yes! You bet, in spades. That being said, it may not be the same life you have been leading. I surely am transformed by the experience of this disease, and for the better. You will hear similar sentiments from many people who have faced RA and are doing what it takes to manage their symptoms. Like them, you can have an active life of regular exercise, good eating, and some relaxation practice—perhaps yoga, meditation, tai chi, quiet reflective strolls. And you will be assembling and managing a team of people who will be informing and supporting your wellness.

Among those who do poorly are those who expect to get well from a pill, who leave their fate in the hands of a doctor, or who cling to a stress-inducing lifestyle. The situation comes down to whether or not your wellness is the most important thing in your life. If it is, and you act on that, then the good life follows.

Who gets arthritis?

Although arthritis has been thought of as a disease of the elderly, people of all ages are affected. Among the two million Americans and over fifty million people worldwide with RA, three times more women than men are affected. The onset of the disease is increasingly more common with age, peaking in the middle years. Those with family members who have RA are at some increased risk, but a study of identical twins (people with the same genes) showed that when one twin had RA, the other twin did not necessarily get it, although the risk, 15 to 20 percent, is higher than for other siblings. (See Month 8.)

How long does it take to feel better?

The answer varies widely among individuals. Some disease-modifying drugs take months to take effect, and it is possible that you may try more than one before you find the best for you. Your doctor may offer a "bridge" drug to take in the meantime. It can take time to adjust to dealing with the disease, to realize the need to pace your day, incorporate rest, eliminate chronic stressors, or begin to participate in groups or classes. It is possible to feel overwhelmed and out of control; you can become depressed and lose the momentum you need to manage a program. You will note the mention of small rewards in this book, ways of enticing you to stick with your program, that have the added benefit of enhancing your brain chemistry and keeping hope alive.

An arthritis support group will put you in touch with others going through a similar process that will help to put it in perspective.

Is there a cure for RA?

The short answer is no, but that word cure, which was never spoken, is now in lively discussion among researchers. The disease and its causes have been elusive because the causes vary among individuals. But the genetic and environmental components are coming to light. The North American Rheumatoid Arthritis Consortium has twelve centers across the country working full time to discover all the genes that influence RA. Many researchers believe that cures will be developed in our lifetimes. Once the genes are identified, genetic reprogramming is one possibility; it is already in lab development.

In the meantime, many people like me are in remission with new combinations of more specifically targeted drugs, together with management programs. Every component is individual, but for those with the patience to explore what is most helpful, RA is manageable.

IN A SENTENCE:

> *The answer to the biggest question we all have is yes, you can live an active and productive life if you have RA.*

learning

Drugs that Modify RA

BEYOND THE analgesics and the NSAIDs are other drugs used in the treatment of rheumatoid arthritis, as well as a less frequently used blood process:

Corticosteroids relieve inflammation, but do not modify the progression of the disease.

Disease-modifying antirheumatic drugs (DMARDs) do influence the disease.

Biologic response modifiers (BRMs), the newest drugs, are specifically targeted to the disease.

Protein-A immunoadsorption is a blood-filtering process.

This is a partial list intended as an explanation of drug categories. Among the examples, the absence of a particular drug does not comment on its efficacy. As always, drug choices are made by you with your doctor.

Corticosteroids

Steroid refers to a wide category of substances defined by chemical structure. The category includes cholesterol, estrogen, and the anabolic steroids in the sports news. The steroids used to treat RA are corticosteroids, like prednisone. They are synthetic drugs closely related to cortisol, a hormone that is naturally produced in the adrenal gland. Corticosteroids act on the immune system by blocking the production of substances that trigger allergic and inflammatory actions, such as **prostaglandins**.

The introduction of cortisone for RA treatment fifty years ago was considered a medical miracle. Over the years, the cumulative side effects for many became greater than the benefits.

Balancing gains versus risks in taking corticosteroids is a seesaw. They are powerful drugs that act quickly to reduce swelling and inflammation, although they do not halt the progression of the disease. They have beneficial uses, but potential side effects need to be considered with great respect. For those reasons, steroids are usually prescribed in low doses or for short durations.

People on higher doses or who take it for an extended time can have a Michelin-man look, their puffy faces caused by water retention. They are at risk of high blood pressure, thinning of the skin and easy bruising, adrenal suppression, cataracts, diabetes, osteoporosis, and neurological problems—and that is a partial list.

It is important to avoid self-regulation of dosage. If you are on this drug for a long time, a doctor needs to monitor a gradual reduction to permit the adrenal glands to resume natural cortisol production; eliminating doses too quickly can result in a life-threatening drop in cortisol. The body can exhibit withdrawal symptoms caused by removing the drug after longtime use. I have been through this process, and it was very extended. I have also met a person with serious permanent damage to her health from taking herself off cortisone abruptly.

Why, you may be wondering, would you even consider taking such a drug? Corticosteroids offer rapid, systemic relief as a "bridge therapy" for brief periods before other drugs become effective. Expert rheumatologists use occasional low doses of corticosteroids for short times, and they also use them to inject a flaring joint. Steroid injections, like a short course of prednisone taken by mouth, have few side effects. They can result in a pronounced reduction of inflammation. Repeated injections in the same area can cause damage, however, but you and I do not need to pitch in the World Series. One rheumatologist suggested that I could have three such injections in my lifetime, one for the wedding of each of my sons.

If you do take a corticosteroid, it is helpful to take adequate calcium and vitamin D supplements to protect against the possibility of osteoporosis. Note that the steroids sold by brand name are much more expensive than prednisone.

DMARDs: Methotrexate

Unlike the drug categories listed above, disease-modifying antirheumatic drugs (DMARDs) can, as their name implies, affect the course of RA. Starting early with such specialized medication helps control inflammation and avoid joint deterioration. It is easier to control the disease in its early stages, and more difficult, as one rheumatologist put it, to get the horse back in the barn. Your choice of DMARD and whether or not you begin with a combination DMARD and biologic will depend upon your doctor, you, and your insurance rules.

The most often prescribed DMARD is **methotrexate**. The drug was originally used for cancer in much higher doses. For RA, it is taken once a week at a low dose. It takes some time to have an effect, but like other DMARDs, efficacy lasts for a number of years. It works as a decoy, fitting into the same cell receptor as folic acid and diminishing the activity of the immune system. It is often prescribed in combination with a biologic drug.

It is recommended that folic acid is taken with methotrexate, that alcohol intake be eliminated or extremely moderate, and that you be monitored with regular blood tests. Methotrexate cannot be taken in pregnancy. For some people, side effects are lessened if it is administered intramuscularly.

At the low weekly doses used to treat rheumatoid arthritis, serious side effects are not common. Those most often listed are upset stomach, chest pain, mouth sores, sore throat, hair loss—some of which subside. A list of the rare side effects (boils, convulsions, paralysis) is included with your medication; it's as though your airline ticket would mention the rate of motion sickness and crash fatalities. If you do develop a side effect or suspect that you have a drug allergy, contact your doctor.

Other DMARDs

Among the DMARDs, gold compounds were once commonly used, but are used less often now. It is known that gold compounds decrease the number of inflammatory white blood cells in the joint fluid (see Month 7 for how the immune system acts in the joint).

Hydroxychloroquine (Plaquenil) was originally a malaria medication. It is one of the best tolerated DMARDs. It may take several months for the drug to take effect, possibly requiring an interim medication. It is often used in combination with other DMARDs, particularly methotrexate. Although regular eye examinations are required, retinal problems are rare and reversible when the drug is stopped. Bright sunlight is not recommended. Other potential side effects include nausea or headache. Monitoring is important, particularly if you have allergies to related drugs or have a retinal abnormality.

Leflunomide (Arava) was developed for RA and is reported to reduce symptoms. Possible side effects include chest congestion, painful urination or breathing, hair loss, and headache. Because the drug may persist in the body for up to two years, it is not appropriate for women who may become pregnant or for men who wish to father a child.

Sulfasalazine was designed in 1938 specifically for RA, which at that time was believed to be caused by bacteria. It appears to help retard progression of RA both alone and in combination by suppressing the immune system. It has an antibacterial agent (sulfapyridine) and an anti-inflammatory agent (salicylic acid). Its side effects may include nausea, headache, and sensitivity to sunlight. Monitoring is important, particularly if you are allergic to sulfa drugs or aspirin. The medication takes three or four months to take full effect.

Biologic response modifiers (BRMs)

[We have entered] a new era of safer and more effective treatments for arthritis. We are still in the early stages, but it has begun. It is the result of fifteen years of unprecedented progress in our understanding of the basic biology of the rheumatic diseases. A clearer picture of those mechanisms has led to new ideas about how to treat these diseases. Almost all of the new therapies have very precise targets on which they are focused. It is a dramatic change from all previous arthritis therapies, which generally were discovered without a full understanding of how they worked or even why they worked.
—DR. DAVID WOFSY, PROFESSOR OF
MICROBIOLOGY AND IMMUNOLOGY AT THE
UNIVERSITY OF CALIFORNIA AT SAN FRANCISCO

The words "breakthrough" and "remission," once rarely spoken when talking about arthritis treatment, are present-day realities. Not everyone responds to the new biologic drugs, but as many as two-thirds do.

BRMs can stop disease progression and, in many cases, mine included, initiate a long-lasting remission. They often work for people for whom other therapies have failed, and some health insurance plans restrict use to these patients. The biologics are often prescribed in combination with a standard DMARD, usually methotrexate.

The biologic drugs are genetically engineered versions of naturally occurring molecules that bind cytokines, proteins produced in the immune response that cause inflammation. (See Month 7 for an explanation of how the immune system works and how it functions with RA.) These proteins produce messages that determine whether certain immune cells, T cells, will differentiate into cells that promote or diminish inflammation. Although there are as many as twenty-four different cytokines that play a role in RA, one, **tumor necrosis factor alpha (TNF-alpha)**, is targeted by the biologics adalimumab (Humira), etanercept (Enbrel), and infliximab (Remicade). Another cytokine, **interleukin-1 (IL-1)** is targeted by anakinra (Kineret).

Biological drugs must be infused intravenously (Remicade) or injected (Enbrel, Humira, Kineret). The molecules in biologic drugs are too large to be delivered any way but by injection. You will be taught to do the injections. Any squeamishness I had about poking myself with a needle has long since been outweighed by the quality of life I have regained. The drugs are very expensive, prohibitively so for many, even with insurance. Getting a prescription will depend upon your doctor, health care plan, and your decision. Because the biologic drugs are so new, the long-term effects are not known. Side effects that have been observed include redness at the injection site and susceptibility to infection. In general, the drugs are well tolerated.

Another rheumatologist at the University of California stated that the biologics are over-rated and observes that, with the exception of fatigue, methotrexate relieves symptoms well in her patients.

Dr. John Klippel, the medical director of the Arthritis Foundation, calls the arrival of the BRMs "the beginning phases of a biologic revolution." Researchers say that future agents may be less expensive and could be taken orally.

Protein-A immunoadsorption

This treatment filters immune substances from the blood. It was approved by the FDA in 1999 for people who don't respond to other therapies. The procedure, similar to kidney dialysis, takes about two hours and is done weekly for twelve weeks. Only one-third of patients respond to the treatment, and those patients reported that it took a full course of treatment to see benefit. Most commonly observed side effects include flu-like symptoms.

Interestingly, in the data gathered by the Iowa Women's Health Study (see Month 8), among RF-positive patients, who would be at higher risk for developing RA, a lower percentage of those who had had a blood transfusion in surgery developed the disease. There seems to have been an immunomodulatory effect that lasted years. The odds of improvement rely on the donor and recipient having at least one particular risk gene in common and a mismatch for the other one—a situation that mimics the immunologic mechanism active in pregnancy. (See Month 10 for an explanation of RA in pregnancy.)

Drugs are used in combination

Many rheumatologists are now combining biologics with DMARDs for the best effect. It takes time for some drugs to come to full efficacy, so it can be a lengthy process to arrive at the combination that works for an individual.

That process of trial and error may end when a new field called personalized medicine is further developed. Identifying the cellular specifics of an individual's disease is said to make it possible to know which drug will work best.

IN A SENTENCE:

> Disease modifying drugs, DMARDs, can help control the progress of RA.

FIRST-WEEK MILESTONE

A week ago seems like the dark ages. After seven days you can celebrate a new understanding of rheumatoid arthritis that frees you from many fears. At this point you know:

○ WHAT RA IS AND HOW IT IS DIAGNOSED.

○ IT IS NOT YOUR FAULT.

○ YOU CAN LIVE WELL WITH RA IF YOU ARE AN ACTIVE PARTICIPANT IN YOUR PROGRAM.

○ SUCCESSFUL MANAGEMENT OF RA IN-CLUDES MORE THAN PRESCRIBED MED-ICATION ALONE; YOU NEED ROUTINE EXERCISE, GOOD NUTRITION, AND RELAX-ATION PRACTICE.

○ STRESS PLAYS A ROLE IN YOUR WELL-BEING, AND IT CAN BE ALLEVIATED.

○ THE TEAM YOU GATHER AROUND YOU WILL PROVIDE HELP IN MANY FORMS, BUT YOU ARE RESPONSIBLE FOR MAINTAINING YOUR OWN PROGRAM.

○ YOU ARE NOT ALONE. YOU HAVE THE CIRCLE
OF UNDERSTANDING FRIENDS AND FAMILY
YOU CREATE AROUND YOURSELF, AS WELL
AS A VAST RA COMMUNITY AVAILABLE TO
YOU IN MANY VENUES, INCLUDING SUPPORT
GROUPS AND ONLINE.

Ways to Effect Change

Oh, my friend, it's not what is taken away that
counts. It's what you do with what you have left.
— HUBERT HUMPHREY

WHAT NEEDS to change with a diagnosis of RA? Nothing, if your program is now in place and working magnificently. You may be the one who can skip this chapter, the one we can all learn from as we struggle to make the life changes that we need to make to manage the disease. The rest of us need to develop some skills to make adjustments in the patterns of our lives and the way we perceive them.

It's a daunting task to change the things we do, let alone change the way we think. Acceptance of our diagnosis is only the beginning. There are many barriers that keep us from modifying behaviors—those within ourselves and those of life circumstances. It seems that one affects the other in a kind of locked bond that needs to be loosened at one end or the other. Change the work schedule to relax the mind and body; relax the mind and body to see the need for changing the work schedule. But if you never examine and let go of a governing belief, in this case that self equals job, then nothing happens to relieve the stress—whether the workday is shortened or not.

Options for changing the exterior conditions of our lives vary widely. One person runs a company and can delegate duties, and another survives on a minimum-wage job or even two. Even when we do make a change, many of us hold to the same habits, double- and triple-tasking in some other arena. As a culture, we suffer from cognitive overload, like mothers of young children who go from work to the next job at home, with no dip in blood pressure.

Time for a change

Perhaps one of the reasons we go to films is to watch people change. On the screen, presto, in an hour and a half you see a new person. Our own change can take years, or for all our good intentions, it never happens at all.

Those of us with this diagnosis are compelled to act within a time frame measured in months to prevent permanent damage to our bodies. Even though we can't pull it off like a movie script, we need to make changes. We have to clear any obstacle in the way of putting our plan into effect.

You have a choice. Choose wellness.

Some skills are basic

The way we think can be a template for success or failure. Optimism alone won't control your RA, but on the other hand, distorted or negative thinking can make it difficult for you to follow your program. These patterns may not always be conscious, but with attention they can be restructured. You will need to communicate with yourself. You will need to adopt strategies for identifying problems and generating solutions.

Commitment to getting well comes with the responsibility to actively participate in your own wellness. The writer Nancy Etchemendy says that she has to recommit to wellness every day. She says that the first step is to become aware of the moment when you are choosing between contributing to your wellness and some other obligation. You don't always make the choice that will help you, but becoming conscious of how you make these decisions is the first step in effecting change.

Problem solving is a coping skill

Outlining obvious, simple steps may seem insulting to your intelligence, but remember that this is in large part a monologue addressed to myself as I was diagnosed. I include it because I repeatedly find myself stuck and having to go back to this process.

If you are feeling stress, write down the things that are bothering you. Choose just one at a time to work on. Consider the problem in a broad perspective, looking at it from different angles. (Picture what would happen if you solve the problem one way or another.) A support group is an excellent venue for this, because it can be hard to see through our own filters. Choose a plan of action to turn the situation to your benefit.

Changing the way you think

> *If you can't change your fate, change your attitude.*
>
> — AMY TAN

Cognitive psychology teaches that people do have choices: they can change their lives; they can change the way they think. When you change the way you look at things, the things you look at change.

We didn't create an autoimmune disease with thought. (Various contributing factors are discussed in Day 2 and Month 8.) But state of mind affects muscle tension, sleep, fatigue, and isolation—all of which contribute to depression, a state in which pain is amplified. Moreover, we know through studies that the immune system can become overactivated in response to chronic stressors. Major life events have been shown to have less negative effect on the immune system than repeated stress. Most important, in studies quoted by Dr. Jerome Groopman of Harvard, the *perceived* controllability of the stressors had the greatest influence on the immune response.

Evaluating stressors

Listen to your body. It is the best source of information about the stress you feel.

You may be better off relaxing or exercising before you take on a situation that is disturbing you. A friend working as a consultant was tense after a disturbing meeting; he found an empty room and went through a tai chi set until he was calm enough to proceed with his work.

It may be easier to avoid or deny a situation, so make an appointment with yourself to confront it. That appointment might best be kept with a group or with a counselor.

Underlying a problem may be a belief that is not serving you (*I can't ask anyone to finish this task*). You may need to have a conversation with yourself (*Is it worth my fatigue and pain to do this? Will the consequences be dire if it's not done? Why do I not want to ask for help?*).

Sometimes our stress stems from a belief that is true (*It's not fair that I am the one in my family to have RA*). Even though it's true, there is no value in holding on to it. Usefulness trumps righteousness.

The way we filter our perceptions

We create filters to experience the world, otherwise it would be too much information to process. Changing a filter can yield a surprising result. I have come to call it the Barn Phenomenon after such a filter-lift of my own. My husband, about to build a barn, asked me to let him know when I saw a barn design that I liked. I told him that I never see barns. But then, along familiar stretches of highway, it seemed that I saw barns everywhere, and I had never noticed.

A filter can distort your perception (*There are no barns here*). A distortion pulled out into the light can reveal a different picture (*Whoa, there are barns I never noticed*). But down in the dark of the psyche, it can block the foresight you need for your own well-being (*I can't choose a barn design because I never see barns*). Common distortions of thought have been listed by Dr. David Burns, now at the Stanford University Medical Center; (I have added examples):

All or nothing thinking. (Now that I have RA, I'll never have a life.) Overgeneralization. (Everybody thinks I'm letting them down because I don't do as much as I used to.)

Mental filter. (A friend does not call; I'm sure he is angry) when in reality, he is out of town.

Disqualifying the positive. (My symptoms improve. I'll never get totally well.)

Jumping to conclusions. (I feel tired. I have the most destructive type of RA.) Magnification or minimization. (I couldn't drive for the class trip. I'm not a good mother.)

Emotional reasoning. (I don't feel like doing anything. I can't do anything.)

Should statements. (I should exercise, eat less, meditate.)

Labeling and mislabeling. (I am a lazy loser.)

Personalization. (It's my fault that the family can't go to the beach.)

Self-talk can be changed

Our filters are an unconscious, ingrained part of us, often narrated by the little voice on our shoulder, like Jiminy Cricket. What we say to ourselves can govern our ability to function—keeping us going or bringing us down. Self-talk is a powerful tool. Negative talk can worsen pain, depression, and fatigue. If there are demons within us, they are our own self-defeating messages.

Just as negative self-talk is learned, positive self-talk can be learned. To make these messages work for instead of against your RA program, begin by paying attention to what you say to yourself and take note of the negative messages. Changing statements takes awareness and practice. Tune in, especially when things don't go your way. Note how you categorize these events—as passing incidents or as signs of persistent bad luck; with acceptance or anger. Be aware of situations that you replay in your mind, and what commentary you play with them. Remember that the same physical response that took place with the stressor is reactivated with the replay; you collect ongoing residuals.It takes time and practice to replace negative narratives. First, you have to come to awareness. Then take a moment to reword the message. *(Nothing I can do will make me better; I'll find some way to improve today, however small.)*

If this is beginning to sound like a lobotomy, bear in mind that turning all of your available power in the direction of your wellness will not drain your life of passion. I invite you to meet people like Nancy Etchemendy and Carol Eustice through their Web sites. (See the Resources section for Web addresses.)

Identify the triggers and process the thought

Awareness of negative or distorted thinking can be alerted by identifying triggers, situations that set it off. When you choose to begin a changed behavior, for example starting to exercise, observe what thoughts get in your way. They come in various forms—perceptions (*I have no time*), emotion (*I don't feel like I can do it*), environment (*my room is too cluttered for exercise*), physical (pain, stiffness), social (*I don't like to work out alone*).

As these patterns appear, you can dissect them and argue yourself out of each barrier. Make a note when they show up:

Situation: I don't feel well enough to exercise.
Automatic thought: I give up; I'll never be able to do it, anyway.
Triggers: Perceptual (I'm not an athlete), emotional (I can't cope).
Distortion: Overgeneralizaton, magnification, jumping to conclusions.
Reappraisal: I know that it is difficult to predict my energy level, and it may take time to balance exercise and rest. I'll break up the workout into shorter periods and start with range-of-motion for fifteen minutes in the morning when I'm less fatigued. I could use a gradual program and will call a physical therapist.

Think of this process as a necessary routine, like brushing your teeth or taking out the garbage; you are getting rid of the plaque and trash of the mind. Just because a thought appears, it doesn't mean that you have to keep it. Learn to see negative events as passing and manageable. That outlook will allow you to become more actively involved in your own care. With a change in perspective, the same threatening diagnosis can be a catalyst for change.

IN A SENTENCE:

> You can change patterns of thinking that interfere with your successful management of your RA.

learning

Leaving Behind Emotional Baggage

Communication: *telling it like it is*

Making a plan means, in practical terms, effective communication with your team and with yourself. You may be good at communication, but the contents are still new. In addition, you may find yourself awash with feelings that come out in unexpected ways.

You can distance those close to you with the anger and resentment that may well up in you when you are dealing with RA. It's best to face the feelings and identify the source. Often, with what you know now, you can use facts to dispel the fear that underlies the feelings: RA is a manageable disease, and you can do it.

Still, communicating can be hard when you are tired or confused. If you are a person who is direct, good. Tell it like it is, but don't take it out on those around you. It's not your fault that you have RA, and it's not theirs, either.

Listening and expressing your feelings with regard for the other person will go farther than an emotional outburst. Test your assumptions by discussing them. Acknowledge the other person's point of view. Paraphrase what you hear to be sure you understand. Use "I" statements rather than "you" statements to diffuse blame. The infusion of kindness into a conversation allows people to relax and be more straightforward. Intellectual qualities are less strongly tied to happiness than values like loving kindness.

Nobody knows the trouble I've seen

Demanding or complaining will cause people to pull away from you in an effort to avoid the unpleasantness. Simply communicating your experience is all you need to do. What is happening for you is so real and so absorbing that it is easy to assume that it must be obvious to everyone around you. But no one knows until you communicate.

Stay connected to people. It will buoy your spirits, distract you from self-absorption, and add to their lives.

The role of forgiveness

> Before you embark on a journey of revenge, first dig two graves.
>
> —Confucius

Holding a grudge can do more than occupy your mind with a feeling of helplessness. It can trigger a stress response in the body that can have a negative impact on your arthritis and your health in general. When you mentally replay situations in which you felt hurt, the body reacts as though the event were happening again. Stress hormones are secreted, causing systemic consequences to the immune system as well as to neurological functions, including memory. One study showed that the level of cortisol, a hormone related to impaired immune function, increased in people asked to think about a problem relationship. (The toxicity of chronic stress is further discussed in Day 2.)

For centuries, religious teachings of many faiths have taught forgiveness as a virtue. Now there is scientific evidence that the act of forgiveness benefits our health. Giving up resentment or anger creates measurable positive changes in your body, including lower blood pressure and heart rates.

"In a way, the most selfish thing you can do for yourself is to forgive other people," wrote Dr. Dean Ornish. When you forgive, you take responsibility for your happiness, rather than give it up to the person who hurt you. Forgiveness not only reduces the physical effects of stress, but it also strengthens social relationships—known to enhance health.

Forgiveness is not an acceptance of hurtful behavior, a pretense that nothing happened, or an excuse for the other person. It does not require repression of anger or feelings of being violated, and it does not even require contact with the offender, although you do need to clear things up directly if it is someone who will remain close to you. It could mean ending an abusive relationship in the best way possible. It is not something you can do before you are willing.

It's hard to let go of a wounded feeling, but it is a learned skill. You can practice on the freeway, dispensing forgiveness to rude drivers. Once you can deal with strangers, take on the weightier grudges. There are stages in the process—examining negative thought, acknowledging that it's time to move on, gaining perspective on the situation by considering the other person's view, deciding to get out of the loop, releasing the emotion. Refocusing how you think about what has happened is a technique that psychologists call narrative repair.

In a study at Duke University, patients suffering pain went through an eight-week course in a traditional Buddhist meditation used to transform anger into compassion. The control group was unchanged at the end of the period, but those doing the practice had significantly less pain and anxiety. You can process forgiveness with the help of friends or a therapist. Some do it through prayer. And you can turn your power to forgive on yourself.

The biology of hope

Positive belief and expectation, the comforted feeling that comes when you project a positive future, can alter neurochemistry. These emotions, best summed up as hope, can trigger the release of endorphins in the brain, mimicking the effects of morphine and blocking pain signals. Emotions alone have not been proven to dictate outcome, but hopefulness does influence well-being.

Educating yourself about RA will show you that you have options, and you will acquire a sense that you can have some control over your diagnosis. Hope gives you clear-eyed courage to meet your circumstances.

Count your blessings with your blood pressure

I thought of counting one's blessings as a homey, quaint example of a cross-stitched maxim. With all that we have learned about the reward and trust circuits in the brain, it makes sense that such an exercise would have positive effects.

Sonja Lyubomirsky, a sychologist at the University of California at Riverside, studied various kinds of mood boosters, with a grant from the National Institutes of Health (NIH). One was a diary in which participants noted things for which they were thankful. The controls reported little change in mood, but those who kept the gratitude journal reported increased satisfaction with their lives. In one exercise, called The Three Blessings, each day the subjects recorded three things that went well and why. They were reported to feel better months later. This does not seem like hard science, but at the University of California at Davis, the psychologist Robert Emmons found that such gratitude exercises affect physical health by raising energy levels, and, for some, relieving pain and fatigue.

So tonight, fall asleep counting your blessings—starting with the gift of your improving health that you are giving to yourself.

Turn outward

Our illness can become an obsession if we allow ourselves to withdraw from others. Reaching out to support others is as important as receiving help, and perhaps more emotionally beneficial. It can lift your sense of well-being to feel useful. There are a lot of ways you can be present for others, even when you are not feeling your best. Sometimes what someone needs is a patient listener. And often, you need to give to another person before that person can give back.

Changes in family dynamics

Teach what you have learned to your friends and family. Most of them are as much in the dark as you were and will be grateful to understand what is going on.

Any change in a family can cause unexpected feelings. A family is an organism. Change in an individual changes the family dynamic; your illness affects everyone else.

Your mate or children may need to take over more responsibility, at home or financially. Children learn that you are no longer playing horse or baseball or driving on field trips. Everyone knows that a flare can cancel your plans, but they may be confused.

RA can be hard on relationships, especially close ones. Your mate may have fallen in love with a wilderness explorer and ended up with someone who has trouble walking up the front stairs. You may be reconsidering your plans to have children. And one person with RA said she hardly thought about sex for a couple of years. All relationships change over time, and it is important to keep an ongoing open dialogue, even without chronic disease. It is even more important to do so with RA, because those close to you cannot know what you are experiencing.

You're not making pancakes? They may just be pancakes for you, but for another member of the family, they may be symbols of love in a Sunday morning ritual. You may not realize that a young child can be afraid that you are dying or that he is responsible for your illness. I was bedridden with severe RA, and my young sons experienced the loss in their lives as a kind of death. There are repercussions to these feelings if left unexplored, and it is wise to head them off early.

RA will change your family. If you communicate openly about it, acknowledging that the expression of hurt and frustration is as important as the expression of love and happiness, the changing dynamic can strengthen your bonds.

Above all, don't isolate yourself. The support of your family and friends will make a difference in your well-being.

Counseling

> I had the blues
> because I had no shoes
> until upon the street
> I met a man who had no feet.
>
> —ANCIENT PERSIAN SAYING

When the writer Nancy Etchemendy had given up hope for her condition, she went to a therapist who specialized in chronic conditions. She found her complaints reframed when she entered the room and discovered that the therapist was paraplegic. His ability to manage a good life and the guidance he provided permitted her to take control of her own life.

Such a cacophony of emotion comes with this diagnosis that it is not easy to be one's own guide. So many psychological filters are invisible to us until they are pointed out. Fear can turn to anger, and those closest to us can suffer. It is a wise person who reaches out for help.

The old prejudice against counseling as being for people who are mentally ill no longer stands in your way if you need help. Well-meaning family and friends are not adept at picking out distorted patterns of thinking that can impede your progress. Choose from individual counseling, family counseling, group counseling or educational groups in stress management and relaxation. Psychiatrists, psychologists, social workers, family counselors, priests, ministers, and rabbis can be helpful.

"If I had one thing to say to a newly diagnosed person, I'd say go to a counselor, get psychological help," writes Nancy.

Join an RA support group

With few people around you with an understanding of what you are experiencing, an RA support group gives you the sense that you are not alone. It offers up a mirror for your perceptions and can provide creative solutions you had not considered.

One woman in a group said she could not multitask anymore. Another one reminded her that managing her illness is its own job, that she is already multitasking, and that's why she can't take on as many things as she used to do. A small observation, but it is another piece of a larger picture that is built bit by bit.

Most groups are well moderated. Occasionally, I read, a group can become a complaint-fest, a group distortion that you can do without. Contact your local Arthritis Foundation office for a list of support groups or self-help courses in your area, and choose one that feels right for you.

IN A SENTENCE:

> *Making a plan requires you to turn both inward and outward with skills that can be learned in counseling.*

Exercise and RA

> *If I'm feeling down and out, the one thing that I*
> *know that's going to get me going is exercise.*
> —DR. ALICE DOMAR,
> HEAD OF THE HARVARD MIND/BODY
> CENTER FOR WOMEN'S HEALTH

Exercise and RA: pick up thy bed and walk

It was once common for a person with rheumatoid arthritis to be consigned to a hospital for two or three months of bed rest. The belief then was that movement was harmful to the joints. Rest did produce some pain relief, but the price of inactivity was physical deterioration. Numerous studies have now shown that not just exercise, but vigorous exercise, is an essential tool in managing RA.

In a study of 5,700 older people with arthritis at Northwestern University near Chicago, inactive adults had twice the risk of functional decline. A Dutch study followed 300 RA patients, median age fifty-four, with half of them in an intensive exercise program. Biweekly one-hour sessions included flexibility routines for warm-up and cool-down; strength training; aerobic activities such as bicycling; and sports including badminton, volleyball, soccer, and basketball. Not only did those in the exercise group improve in functional ability and physical capacity, they felt more optimistic and capable of coping. The benefit of exercise was found to be the greatest in early RA. A recent Finnish study shows that strength training benefits people with RA without increasing disease activity or pain. The American College of Rheumatology recommends regular participation in dynamic exercise.

Not everyone has gotten the message. Another Dutch study found some rheumatologists and more physical therapists still working under the old myth, and recommending rest over movement. You will even find newer books on arthritis exercise with benign programs, as though the disease would be exacerbated by repeated movement. The Arthritis Foundation has taken a stand on the matter, so to speak, by putting on a yearly three-mile walk each May in many American cities to raise both awareness and funds for research.

Still, exercise was discussed in only half the office appointments with rheumatologists studied by researchers at the Harvard School of Public Health. Although you will need your doctor's guidance, the impetus to start an exercise program will come from you.

When we are in pain, the old way is seductive: just crawl into bed and pull the covers up. Both our muscles and our psyches contract, and we tend to withdraw into a vicious cycle of inactivity and growing pain. I know about this; I did it. Although my RA has been in remission for over five years, I have just learned that I will need shoulder replacement surgery. Why the shoulder, which was never one of the joints that was inflamed when I was sick, and why now? The disease is systemic, and all the joints deteriorate when RA is not controlled; weakened cartilage and ligaments can give out much later. I want to be encouraging here, but real optimism is based in fact. I'm here to tell you that you have to move, and you'll feel and be better for it.

Even so, it seems counterintuitive that the thing that will help the most is the thing we are the least inclined to do. It feels as though exercise will use up what little energy we have. What's true is that exercise increases energy. The ways that you can save energy by pacing, resting, organizing, and prioritizing are discussed elsewhere in this book (Months 5 and 11), but saving energy by not exercising is like drinking water from a mirage.

The benefits of exercise

Exercise may not be a cure, but it can prevent some diseases and lessen the effects of others, like RA. Its benefits make it the ideal health enhancer. Not only does it help control RA symptoms, it contributes to overall health and a sense of well-being. If you look at taking care of your body as if it were a business, exercise has the best cost-benefit ratio of any component in your management plan.

A program that includes elements of flexibility exercise, strength training, and aerobic activity—like the one in the Dutch study—is both safe for your joints and full of reward. Each element of your program will bring different benefits. Together, your exercise program:

Improves muscle mass. Muscle supports health, vitality, and independence. Most people lose about a quarter pound of muscle every year starting in their late thirties until, at eighty, they have lost a third of their muscle mass. Aging plays some role in this process, called **sarcopenia**, but it is not the only factor; a sixty-five-year-old woman who has been strength training and doing aerobic exercise for a year is biologically much more like a forty-year-old woman who is not exercising. If the forty-year-old had an exercise regime, she would be like a sedentary twenty-year-old. For those of us with RA, strength training increases joint stability and helps to prevent deformities.

Reduces pain. Without exercise, muscles can get out of balance. For example, the muscles in the knee, the hamstrings, and the quadriceps, can drift out of alignment, adding to the pain caused by RA. Also, strengthened muscles can better absorb the impact of walking or standing. In a Tufts University study of people with arthritis of the knee, strength training brought a 45 percent reduction in pain. Other research has shown that regular aerobic exercise can reduce joint swelling in RA.

Reduces fatigue and improves stamina. Exercise improves the distribution of oxygen throughout your body, giving you more available energy. Aerobic exercise builds endurance and strengthens your cardiovascular system.

Can reduce inflammation. Studies suggest that exercise suppresses the inflammatory process by altering the causative enzymes called cytokines. A study cited in *Arthritis Today* magazine of healthy men aged sixty-five to seventy-four concluded that the more physically active they were, the fewer inflammatory chemicals their cells produced. Inflammation that affects joints affects arteries, too, increasing blood pressure. Movement increases cardiovascular health.

Reduces stress, fights depression. Several studies have shown that the physiological stress response diminishes with exercise. A reduction in depression was shown in a ten-week supervised strength training program at Tufts University. Other studies have shown reductions in depression with aerobic exercise. A study in *The British Journal of Sports Medicine* found that walking thirty minutes a day boosted moods in depressed patients faster than antidepressants did. A study at the California State University at Long Beach showed that the more steps people took during the day, the better their moods were. It appears that exercise decreases muscle tension and anxiety.

Benefits lungs and heart. Exercise strengthens the heart muscle, lowering blood pressure and heart rate. University of Pennsylvania researchers found that moving enough to increase blood flow stimulates an anti-inflammatory response in the cells of blood vessels, helping to keep arteries open. A report from *The Physicians' Health Study* showed than men who lifted weights at least thirty minutes a week had a reduced risk of heart disease. Aerobic exercise increases lung capacity and circulation. Exercise is also known to lower cholesterol. Heart and lung problems are complications associated with RA, so the influence of exercise is welcome news for us.

Improves the quality of sleep. The Tufts strength training study also showed improvements in sleep patterns. It follows that a good night's sleep improves mood and, in the chain of events that influences our health, makes us more likely to follow through on our program.

Can help control weight. Exercise can burn calories to help you control your weight and relieve stress on your joints. Muscle is the metabolic engine in your body; it burns more calories than fat, so as your muscle mass increases, your metabolic rate goes up. If you are active and you don't lose weight with your program, consider the value of all of the other health benefits. If you are motivated, increase time exercising a little. People burn calories at different rates and exercise intensity varies, so it may take more than thirty minutes of daily exercise to control your weight. The RA factor aside, overweight people who are fit by cardiovascular measurement have death rates at half those of people who are not fit and at normal weight, according to Dr. Stephen Blair, who researches the relationship between living habits and health at the Cooper Institute. So consider weight control an extra bonus from exercise.

Increases flexibility, balance, posture, overall coordination. Range-of-motion exercises increase flexibility. Aerobic exercise increases oxygen to the brain, from where it is sent to muscles, sharpening reaction time and improving balance.

Improves bone density. In a Finnish study of early RA, bone mineral density was maintained with exercise and remained constant five years later. A study at the Mayo Clinic found that a group with two years of strength training showed measurable improvement in bone density six years later—with fewer than half the spinal fractures of the control group. The Tufts study also showed improvement in bone density. Apart from RA, during each year after menopause, a woman typically loses 1 percent of her bone mass. Exercise creates a pull on the bones, stimulating bone density and lowering the risk of osteoporosis. It improves bone calcium levels as well.

Maintains cartilage and possibly promotes cartilage formation. Cartilage, as well as bone and ligaments, can deteriorate with active RA disease. Healthy cartilage is nourished by synovial fluid in the joints. Certain molecules within the cartilage help to regulate the slow movement of the fluid, acting as a kind of pump so that there is always a smooth, moist cartilage surface. Motion and weight-bearing exercise compress the joints and press oxygen and nutrients into the cartilage. Lack of use of the joint reduces the effectiveness of the pumping mechanism. There are no blood vessels in the cartilage, so its health depends on activity that gives it nourishment from the synovial fluid. Some preliminary studies suggest that cartilage formation increases with strength training. In any case, it is important for maintaining cartilage.

Improves digestion. A moving body gets the bowels moving, speeding the passage of food through the intestines.

Reduces risk of type 2 diabetes. It is known that exercise can lower blood sugar. The Tufts study cited above found improved glucose metabolism with strength training.

Slows mental decline. In a study at the University of California at San Francisco, age-related mental decline was lower in a group of women who walked 2.5 miles per day. In a University of Virginia study, men aged seventy-one to ninety-three who walked more than a quarter mile each day were found to have half the incidence of dementia and Alzheimer's.

Bolsters confidence. The Tufts study showed an increase in confidence with strength training. Even studies that are inconclusive regarding improvement of RA symptoms, such as several studies about tai chi for example, all report an increase in a feeling of empowerment or well-being among those who exercise. It stands to reason that a release of tension that improves mood, helps sleep, promotes alertness, and decreases pain would also increase self-image.

What if you don't exercise?

You probably have gathered enough reasons to start an exercise program. But lots of things come up, and it's hard to get around to it; I am a master of this kind of procrastination, so I'm not pointing any fingers. And some of us just don't much like exercise.

The Arthritis Foundation points out that few people realize how dangerous a sedentary life can be, citing experts who believe that it is as much a risk to your health as smoking a pack of cigarettes a day. If you have RA, the pain and stiffness that come with the disease can take you into a downward cycle: You are in pain; you stop moving; your muscles, including your heart, weaken; you become stiffer, more sore, and more fatigued than before. There are other risks as well:

Hypertension, or high arterial blood pressure. One of the major risk factors for hypertension is a lack of physical activity. In addition, people with RA may be at a greater risk for hypertension from the advancement of the disease or from some medications.

Loss of flexibility. RA can cause generalized inflammation that restricts mobility and limits daily activities. Exercise is known to help reduce stiffness.

Loss of muscle mass. Because RA can restrict the movement of joints, muscles are not able to fully stretch and contract. As a consequence they atrophy quickly, becoming more susceptible to sprains and less able to support deteriorating joints.

Deterioration of bone. Natural bone loss that takes place with aging, particularly for women, can be stopped with weight-bearing exercise. Active RA can create bone erosion.

Weight gain. It is commonly believed that weight gain is an unavoidable consequence of aging. Most women assume that hormones cause a gain in weight around the time of menopause. It is a self-fulfilling prophecy; most women do gain weight around the time of menopause, but they don't need to, according to the surprising results of a three-year study of over 3,000 women in midlife called the *Study of Women Across the Nation* (SWAN). Researchers found that the women who started or maintained a high level of physical activity through menopause did not gain weight. Those who started exercise during this period lost weight. Weight is an extra burden for people with RA, because it adds stress to the joints.

Loss of cartilage. Exercise promotes the health of cartilage, which is attacked in RA.

Constipation. A sedentary life slows the passage of food through the system.

Fractures. Without exercise, bones become more brittle, making fractures more common.

Diabetes. When muscles aren't used, their cells become resistant to the insulin that the pancreas secretes. More glucose goes into the bloodstream, which can promote diabetes.

Increased stress, heightened pain, and depression. Loss of function from immobility increases stress, which in turn creates muscle tension, leading to increased pain, and so on in a cycle toward depression.

Well, you thought the side effects of the meds were scary. These results of inactivity, called deconditioning, can be reversed with exercise, so let's get moving.

IN A SENTENCE:

Exercise has a profound positive influence on many physical and mental processes important to managing RA and on the general good health that supports it.

learning

Starting an Exercise Program

IF, LIKE ME, you find that it's hard to start exercising, remember that once you couldn't wait to exercise—no matter how far back into your skipping, running, leaping childhood you have to reach. Now is always the best time to begin anew, whatever your age. People at ninety-three who started strength training at Tufts University gained benefit.

For those of us with RA, we of the ticking clock, now really does mean now. Exercise can relieve pain in joints and keep them flexible and well supported. With regular exercise, we are much more likely to stay active. And, if it is sometimes no fun to live with ourselves, think of how it is for those who live with us; the more we move the better we feel. Okay, you say, good idea. The hardest part is starting.

First things first; see a professional

I have taken some wrong turns, and I hope this book can help you avoid them. When my RA was raging, I took to my bed. With my RA in remission, I plunged into exercise on my own and damaged weakened ligaments and atrophied muscle. No matter what the state of your disease, commit to exercise at some level, and make that plan with a professional. Get your physician's approval before you start.

A physical therapist, trained and certified in a range of approaches, can help you set up a program with only a few meetings. It is worthwhile to know correct techniques and precautions; the angle of your body can make the difference between help and harm.

Without expert guidance, you can jar your body, create lack of balance in your core strength, waste your time, or injure yourself by misusing weight machines or cardiovascular trainers. Even your bike needs to be fitted correctly, not only for comfort and efficiency but to avoid injury.

Getting started

You will need to resolve to restructure your day around your most important priority, your health. Easier said than done, but everything you care about—those you love, your work, and the things you want to do—depend on it. It's hard to find the time, but think of it this way: If you exercise, you will have more useful time than you do now. What good is time when you are too fatigued or in pain to do much? A good program will energize you and give you more productive hours—not to mention years of life.

Determine how much time you will set aside each week to start, and formalize it by blocking out the time on your calendar. Give that time first priority and protect it. If that seems self-centered, remind yourself that giving begins with your well-being.

Write your goal in your exercise journal (see Month 2). Start out slowly, creating a routine by linking your workout to a specific time or an activity—before breakfast or lunch or after work—or a time of day when you expect to be flexible and rested. Some people make a contract with themselves. The Arthritis Foundation estimates that it takes twelve weeks for an exercise routine to become a habit, so be patient. I know, I know, so much patience required.

Choosing what you like to do

You will eventually have a program of flexibility, strengthening, and aerobic exercise. There are various ways to lay out your plan, but flexibility or range-of-motion exercises for your arthritic joints will help if they are done every day.

If you choose activities you love to do, you're more likely to stick with them. You'll find your experience of enjoyment particular to you, and you will need to be the gauge of what activities please you. In a wine tasting group, I observed week after week each person's assumption that what he or she perceived was correct. In fact, there was no objectively good wine; opinions differed according to individual preference. When you set up your program, consider your personality: Do you love solitude or do you thrive on company? Are you self-motivated or do you need encouragement? Do you enjoy the out-of-doors or prefer to watch the news from an exercycle? Consider cost: Do you want to spend more to join a gym, less to go to a community center, or take advantage of things you can do for free?

Physical activity simply means movement of the body that uses energy. Being active is a good thing, but don't confuse activity with exercise. Yes, all the steps you take throughout the day will benefit you, as will walking up stairs, bringing in the groceries, taking out the garbage. The more active you are, the better you'll feel. But when it comes to improving your flexibility, strength, and endurance, your daily activities may not be intense enough to increase your heart rate, so you should not count these towards the thirty or more minutes a day that is your goal.

For the health benefits we need, physical activity should be moderate to vigorous. Moderate activity can include bicycling at less than ten miles per hour, light weight training, dancing, yard work, yoga, tai chi, walking at about 3.5 miles per hour. At Columbia University, a study of arthritis patients found that with eight weeks of walking, they experienced a decrease in pain of 27 percent, less need for medication, and an increase in the distance they could walk.

More vigorous activity includes aerobics, freestyle swimming, bicycling at over ten miles per hour, brisk walking at over 3.5 miles per hour, heavy yard work, weight training, rowing, tennis, basketball, volleyball, handball, snowshoeing, golf without a cart, Pilates, dancing, as well as working out on equipment such as elliptical trainers, stair-steps, treadmills, cross-country ski machines, or trampolines. A New York cardiologist, Dr. Mehmet Oz, recommends vigorous sex.

You'll need both weight-bearing and aerobic exercises. Your choices are vast: Dancing? Try line dancing, rock 'n' roll, hip hop, disco, ballroom, folk dancing, square dancing, hula, belly dancing, contra dancing, tango, cha cha, rumba, salsa, tap, ballet, jazz, swing, and so on into your fantasy.

There are different kinds of yoga: Bikram, hatha, Iyengar, yin. And health clubs have spinning (fast exercycling) classes, mind-body cardio classes (newfangled combinations of practices designed to sweat you to serenity) as well as contraptions to exercise every muscle. There is something out there, or at home, for everyone.

If you are reluctant to start because you are in pain, you may prefer water exercise, which reduces stress on your joints. Buoyancy helps support your body while you increase flexibility, increase your heart rate to burn calories, and build cardiovascular health. You can also build muscle strength with water resistance. Find out if the Arthritis Foundation Aquatics Program is available in your area by calling your local office. (See the Resources section of this book.)

Most people find it hard to go it alone and stay motivated, so it's good to buddy up. I once jogged nearby hills alone until a sheriff's warning urged the public to go with partners; the commitment got me out much more regularly. Multiple studies have shown that support from others can help change behaviors. Some experts say that couples who exercise together are more likely to stick to a plan; I can't keep up with my mate, so we go to the gym together and do different things. One friend has been walking before work for years, whether in or out of the mood, with a wake-up call from a colleague. A dog pawing at the door can work, too. A class can give you a feeling of shared goals, as well as a schedule.

Measuring your heart rate

Before you start aerobic exercise, learn to measure your heart rate. The most accurate method is a treadmill stress test, which you want to get if you have been sedentary for a long time or have a history of heart disease. You can buy a heart rate monitor. If you don't have one (I don't), here is another way to find your heart rate:

Put your index finger on the side of your neck between your jaw and collarbone. You can feel your heart beat in the carotid artery. Count for six seconds and add a zero to get your heart rate. (The longer you count, the more accurate the reading: count for thirty seconds and multiply by two.) You can also use the radial artery on the inside of your wrist.

To determine your target heart rate for aerobic exercise, first determine your maximum heart rate. For women, it is 226 minus your age in years; for men, 220—obviously an approximation. You, your doctor, and your physical therapist will decide on the intensity of your training. Use your maximum heart rate to determine your training zone:

> *Warm-up or beginning zone*—Fifty to 60 percent of maximum heart rate. This is the best place to begin a fitness program if you don't have one already. You can use this target later for your warm-up exercises. At this heart rate, you can decrease body fat and cholesterol as well as improve circulation and sleep. About 85 percent of calories burned in this zone are fats.
>
> *Fitness zone*—Sixty to 70 percent of maximum heart rate. At this rate, you have the benefits of the first zone with more calories burned at about the same percentage of fat. You may want to start at below 60 percent, but at that point sustainable gains begin.
>
> *Aerobic zone*—Seventy to 80 percent of maximum heart rate. This rate of exercise is said to increase the size and strength of your heart as well as improve your respiratory system. More calories are burned, with about half from fat.

People who are not endurance athletes gain little additional value when their heart rate goes above 80 percent of maximum. Most programs suggest getting your heart rate up to between 50 to 80 percent of maximum several times a week for twenty minutes or more.

Measuring your BMI

Another measure to take before you begin your program is your **body mass index**; **BMI** is measure of body fat based on height and weight that applies to both adult men and women. To determine your BMI, first measure your height in your bare feet in the morning, because gravity can make you up to half an inch shorter by evening. Sorry, I haven't come up with a trick for weight, once you take your scuba tanks off.

You can calculate your BMI using this formula: BMI equals a person's weight in pounds divided by height in inches squared, multiplied by 703. Huh? You can go to the National Institutes of Health (NIH) National Heart, Lung and Blood Institute site, which will automatically calculate your

BMI when you enter your height and weight: http://nhlbisupport.com/bmi/bmicalc.htm.

The BMI categories are: Underweight, under 18.5; normal, 18.5 to 24.9; overweight, 25 to 29.9; obese, 30 or greater. This does not reflect the state of your fitness; it does not show the difference between fat and muscle, so it may not be accurate for the very muscular or for the elderly with lost muscle mass. It is less useful for people under five feet tall. However, for most people, BMI is a good indicator of whether their weight is a health risk. The Arthritis Foundation emphasizes that even a modest weight loss will reduce the risk of knee damage.

Waist circumference; apples and pears

The location of fat on your body is an indicator of whether you are more likely to develop health problems in addition to RA. If you carry weight around your waist, like an apple, rather than around your hips and thighs like a pear, it is more important for you to address your weight, even if your BMI is below twenty-five and your cholesterol level is low.

Research has shown that stress increases cortisol in the body, which influences the distribution of fat toward the abdomen. This type of fat secretes inflammatory chemicals, worsening swollen joints and increasing risk for heart disease. Weight gain appears to promote a group of risk factors known as metabolic syndrome.

Measure your waist by relaxing and then putting a tape measure firmly but not tightly around your abdomen above your hipbone. A measurement of more than thirty-five inches for women or forty inches for men may indicate a higher disease risk because of the location of the fat.

Exercise equipment

Before you decide to make a substantial investment in exercise equipment, you need to consider that the exercycles on the curbs of most yard sales were once bought in a rush of dedicated enthusiasm. You can buy someone's abandoned dream, but you might be wise to get a program in place before you begin to ornament the family room. It serves only as a discouraging reminder if it is not used.

You can do very handsomely without any of the following, but you may find some of these things useful: Handgrips: soft squeeze balls, handles that press together; Chinese metal balls to rotate in the palm; heart monitor; pedometer; hand-held or wraparound weights; elastic bands known as theraband or theratube; portable player for music or recorded books. I am never so eager to get out and exercise as when I am into a good audio book.

IN A SENTENCE:

> To establish an exercise program, break down the steps into choosing a type of exercise that suits you, establishing an appropriate level of activity, and committing to a schedule.

Specific Exercises for RA

Ease into the right amount of exercise

You will eventually have a program of flexibility, strengthening, and aerobic exercise. There are various ways to lay out your plan, but flexibility or range-of-motion exercises for your arthritic joints will help if they are done every day.

How much is enough? The commonly recommended measure of thirty minutes per day came from the Centers for Disease Control in 1995. The latest Agriculture Department recommendations, called My Pyramid, call for thirty minutes per day to reduce the risk of chronic disease. An additional thirty to sixty minutes per day is recommended to manage weight—a daunting recommendation to the less Spartan of us, who might do nothing in the face of it. (See the Resources section.) Remember, even moderate activity has benefit.

If you are not already fit, start out slowly and build up. Make it fun. Begin with flexibility exercises—stretching that will improve your range of motion and help you perform daily activities. When you are ready, you can move on to weight training and endurance exercises such as bicycling.

Your physical therapist or trainer will suggest increments for building up your program. The two-hour rule is that if you have soreness generated by the workout for more than two hours after a session, it means you need to scale back. If you feel little or no exertion, most trainers advise that you add intensity before you add time.

A good program begins each day, usually in the morning, with range-of-motion exercises. Additional exercise is individually planned and increased according to your ability, starting with, for example:

- O Moderate exercise twice a week for fifteen to thirty minutes, increasing to vigorous before going to three times a week.
- O Short bouts, as long as they add up to thirty minutes two or three times a week—intense enough to raise your heart rate.
- O Strength training fifteen minutes; aerobic exercise fifteen minutes or longer; flexibility cool-down five to ten minutes—two or three times a week.
- O Strength training class once a week, brisk walking once a week, yoga class once a week or a combination of your choice.
- O Daily thirty-minute exercise period alternating between strength and aerobic training.

The five-year Finnish exercise study that stabilized bone density, increased muscle strength, and diminished clinical symptoms in RA patients used a program of flexibility training twice a week, strength training once or twice a week, and aerobic exercise two to three times a week.

Warm-up and cool down

Here is the sadder but wiser voice of experience speaking: Failure to warm up properly cost me a ligament in my knee—a big price for omitting a small thing. Always, always warm up for five minutes or preferably longer before you exercise.

You can use range-of-motion exercises to warm up, and whatever else you do, begin the activity with a lower intensity. Your increasing heart rate will bring warm blood into the muscles and lubricate the joints. The muscles and tendons become more elastic and less prone to injury.

Cooling down after exercise is equally important. Slow down your activity for at least five minutes; some say longer than your warm-up. You may prefer to do most of your stretching after your workout when the warm tissue is more pliant.

Range-of-motion exercise

When I call the dog in the morning, I've learned from her not to be in a hurry. She takes a long, slow stretch of her spine, then flexes each leg back as she draws her neck into an arc and holds it. Our own mammalian bodies have the same need to loosen up when we rise. It feels good.

Range-of-motion or flexibility exercise is the foundation of any program. For RA, it helps reduce stiffness and keep joints mobile for the activities of daily living. Range refers to the normal amount your joints can be moved in various directions, an amount that can be restricted in RA by inflammation or inactivity. These exercises increase movement in muscles, tendons, and ligaments.

The goal is to slightly exceed the restricted movement of the joint. Progress is measured in quarter- or half-inch increments; overambitious pushing can result in injury. Set small goals and celebrate your gains. Flexibility training does not require a day of rest, as strength training does. You can use this phase of your program as a warm-up or cool-down for other exercise. A five- to ten-minute cool-down flushes out the muscles and improves your recovery time.

Moist heat can help you warm up before you stretch, or you can use the shower, hot tub, or sauna as a place to do some range-of-motion. You can also go through much of your stretching in bed in the morning. Flexibility exercises in the evening before sleeping can help morning stiffness. If a joint is too sore to move on its own, move it passively through its range of motion two or three times a day. This will help relieve stiffness and prevent a diminished range.

You can choose from various exercises for this part of your program. The Finnish study that showed increased strength and stabilized bone density in RA patients included stretching for all joints of the upper and lower extremities and neck, ten times for each exercise.

If you haven't exercised for some time, start out with fifteen minutes a day of flexibility exercises, increasing from one or two repetitions of each exercise to ten. At that point, you may be ready to add strengthening and aerobic exercise.

Do these exercises gently. Stretch as far as you can go and hold the position for a few seconds. Don't bob up and down or force it. You will find more in references for exercise programs in the Resources section of this book.

Head and neck. Bend ear to shoulder sequentially on either side, head to chest. Roll your head 360 degrees over your chest and shoulders, and back the other way. Tuck your chin in, hold and release. Move your head up, lengthening your neck.

Shoulders. Do shoulder circles forward and then back. Shrug your shoulders, hold, and lower. Reach your arms forward and then straight up. Put the backs of your hands on your lower back and then slide them up slowly. Put your hands behind your head and then bring your elbows forward.

Spine and hips. Hands on waist, bend forward, back, and to the sides; rotate your hips in a circle; twist your upper body to one side at the waist and then to the other side. Lift each leg to the side. Hold on to the back of a chair and extend each leg behind you; squat slowly, keeping your back straight, then rise up straight onto your toes. Rotate each leg on your heel.

Knees. Raise each knee until your thigh is parallel to the floor, then lower it.

Elbows. Stretch out arm with palm facing you, pull the palm down with the other hand until you feel a stretch, then make a fist and rotate it as though you are opening a door. Hold, and reverse arms.

Hand, wrist, elbows. Hold your elbows to your sides and raise your hands to a 90-degree angle, turning your palms straight up, then down. In the same position, hold your hands with palms facing forward and then lower them until backs of your hands are forward, up and down like the flap on an envelope. Make loose fists, fanning out fingers one at a time so that they are straight, then returning them to the fist one by one. With your hands open, bend your thumbs in and out.

Foot, ankle. Seated, spell out words with your toes—anything you like; the literary foot can try a quote from Robert Browning, "Put forward your best foot." Turn your feet inward, outward, and wiggle your toes.

These are the routines I use every morning in bed before rising:

○ With legs raised straight up, reach hands up as far as possible toward toes, and pull legs as far back overhead as possible.
○ Bring knees to chest with arms laid open straight on bed; roll knees to the side with head turned in opposite direction, stretching the neck. Alternate.
○ Keep knees bent up with feet on bed and arms out to the side; arch back, hold, release.
○ Lie down, keep one knee flexed, and stretch other leg straight, with opposite arm extended straight back to headboard. Alternate.
○ With knees bent, tilt pelvis and sit up partway.

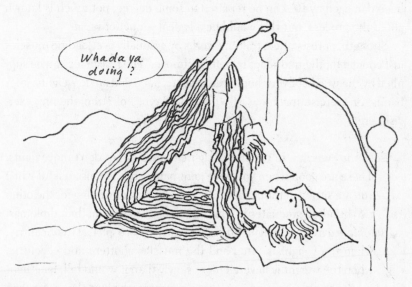

Try range-of-motion exercises in bed before you get up.

In a hot shower I continue:

○ Roll head around 360 degrees on shoulders. Reverse direction.
○ Rotate shoulders in forward circles. Reverse.
○ Stretch arm through full range of motion, including reaching back both below shoulder and above. Repeat with other arm.
○ Clinch fingers into a fist, and release one finger at a time.

Strength training

It is possible to become stronger than you were when you were younger. One study showed that women and men aged seventy-two to ninety-eight could triple their leg strength by doing resistance exercises. Muscle weakness in RA patients was reversed with strength training in a Tufts University study. Strength training also burns fat. Muscle mass is metabolically active tissue that burns about fifty calories per pound, in contrast to fat, which burns two to three calories per pound.

Strength training also helps keep bone density stable by stimulating the cells that make new bone—which is especially important for women, who can begin to lose bone beginning as early as age thirty-five. Bone that has been damaged by RA can be repaired to some degree; not much is known about the process, but this would be a logical venue for repair.

Strength, or resistance, training works by gradually overloading muscles just enough for them to adapt by getting stronger. The resistance can be supplied by the weight of your body, free weights, hand and ankle weights, latex bands, or exercise machines. Two common types of strengthening exercises are:

Isometric exercises, in which you tighten muscles but don't move joints. These are good when you have joint pain. They are also useful while you are sitting in traffic, on hold on the phone, or waiting for the other two hundred graduates in your niece's class to receive their diplomas.

Isotonic exercises—weight lifting, which has two phases: concentric, when the weight is lifted and the muscles shorten, and eccentric, when the weight is lowered more slowly than it would fall, lengthening the muscle. Eccentric exercise may increase blood flow more than concentric, so allow the weight to descend slowly. There is a school of thought that maintains that lowering the weight should be extremely slow, but that has not been proven to be necessary. A single lift of, say, eight seconds could be three seconds to raise, one to pause, and four to lower. The muscle, not gravity or momentum, needs to do the work.

The correct program will provide just enough resistance for your muscles to adapt, not so much that they are sore and stiff the next day. If you have pain, don't start or increase pain medication, because it can interfere with muscle repair and hide signs of your body's tolerance. The point is to strengthen and relieve stress on joints, not to exacerbate it.

Dr. Miriam Nelson of Tufts University has done a number of strength training studies. Her weight-training program is thirty minutes a day. You can download a book from Tufts, *Growing Stronger; Strength Training for Older Adults*, that looks ideal for RA, whatever your age (see Resources).

Many programs alternate muscle groups or strength training days. You can start to build muscle with sessions of twenty to thirty minutes twice a week.

The increase in joint stability that comes with weight-bearing exercise is crucial to the health of an RA patient. In only three months of progressive strength training you can expect an increase in the muscles around your joints. At about that time, depending on the person and the intensity of the workouts, you will experience a metabolic change, with muscle burning more calories than fat. Bone takes longer to respond, but within a year, you should have evidence of more stable bone density. The timing and degree of these changes vary with the individual.

The key in strength training is repeated motion. Be able to do eight to twelve "reps" before increasing the weight or resistance. If you can't do eight, decrease the weight. Progress from easy to hard in intensity for each exercise.

The weight you use can be your own body, as with push-ups or sit-ups; stretch bands that create resistance for pulling or pushing; free weights, hand or ankle weights; exercise machines. You can add weight training by strapping weights to your ankles or wrists when you walk, or you can carry hand weights. Some people find that holding canned goods works fine.

Upper body: Start with light weights and learn to do the lifts correctly— no more than two or three pounds. I do four exercises, done in a standing position, recommended by Kate Lorig in *The Arthritis Helpbook*.
O *The upright row*. Standing, lower the weights in front of you, palms in. Think chicken wings: raise the weights to chest level, elbows out. Lower.
O *Lateral lift*. Arms down to your sides. Think half a snow angel: lift weights, palms down, straight out to shoulder level until arms are parallel to the floor. Lower.
O *Triceps press*. With your hands at your waist and elbows back, bend

forward forty-five degrees and extend weights straight back. Think racing swimmer ready to take off from the block.

○ *Biceps curl.* With arms down at your sides and palms forward, bend at the elbows and bring the weights up to your shoulders. Think holding up a garment to see how it will look.

Core body: Repeat the same curl used as a morning flexibility exercise; lie down with knees bent, feet on the floor. Sit partway up. Repeat.

Lower body (ankle weight can be added):

○ *Leg lifts.* Hold on to the back of a chair and raise your leg straight up and lower. Raise it to the side and lower. Raise it to the back and lower.

○ *Stair steps.* Put one foot on the first stair, straightening it slowly as you bring the other one up. Reverse the process. Change feet. This does more than one might think.

Hands: Use a handled handgrip or a squeeze ball. Slowly squeeze as hard as you can for five to ten seconds. Repeat and switch hands. Increase gradually to thirty seconds, pressing each finger five seconds.

Endurance exercise

When you are ready, add aerobic exercise to your program. Endurance or aerobic exercise uses the large muscles of body in rhythmic, continuous motion, bringing the pulse up to a targeted rate. The purpose, for those of us with RA, is to strengthen the circulatory system so that we pump more blood through the body with each beat, reducing fatigue, controlling weight on joints, improving sleep, reducing depression, and building endurance and stamina. It's a bargain for the investment of your time. Brisk walking, water aerobics, and bicycling are among the most often chosen endurance exercises for people with RA.

Start with a few minutes and work up to a goal, say, thirty minutes five times a week. In the beginning you may prefer to exercise in short bouts adding up to thirty minutes, as long as they are intense enough to raise your heart rate. Begin your workout slowly, building up to your target heart rate and taking your pulse to check it. (How to find it is explained in Week 3.) I don't jog any more, but I still think of exercise as running for my life.

IN A SENTENCE:

> *Your program of three kinds of exercise will begin with range-of-motion, and you will gradually add strength and then aerobic training.*

learning

Other Ways to Exercise

Remember posture

Mother was right when she goaded us to stand up straight—more right than she could have known. With RA, good posture is crucial for minimizing stress on joints. With joint pain, we naturally compensate by putting pressure on the better leg, and that can lead to more painful joint imbalance.

Start with aligning your feet, which has a positive effect on the ankles, knees, hips, and spine. Distribute weight evenly on both feet, keeping them parallel at about shoulder width. It may feel odd, since many people tend to turn their feet outward.

Think of the old image of a string pulling you straight from the top of your head or a plumb bob dropping down to align yourself. You'll find that this stance brings your shoulders back and down, opening your chest and increasing your lung capacity. With your knees straight but not locked, your tailbone slightly under, your shoulders back, you will feel a center of balance that will allow you to lean in any direction and keep your balance.

Exercise and morning stiffness or flares

Most of us with RA have experienced "gelling," a phenomenon caused by the accumulation of fluid in the joint. The fluid is gradually absorbed back into the blood when the joints start moving. A warm bath or shower just after getting up will relax muscles and start the process. Range-of-motion exercises will shorten the period of stiffness. If you need to, use your opposite hand to move a joint through its range.

Flares can be heightened by stress. It is common to put aside exercise when, say, you are bearing down on a deadline, but you can avoid a flare by making the relief of stress the most important motivator for exercise.

You can use an orthotic device or a splint to protect particularly inflamed joints, such as the brace I used on my wrist for a long time. You can also adapt exercises—for example you can do range-of-motion in a chair, holding on to the back of a chair, in the shower, or in bed.

Barriers, distractions, sabotage, and support

I know this subject well, as I went down many back alleyways of procrastination before I got on my way with an exercise program. A few common barriers to starting:

Belief that exercise may be harmful. Let your doctor decide. Some older people are afraid of the rapid breathing and increased heart rate caused by aerobic exercise. Unless there is an underlying medical reason, both are indicators of your body increasing its capacity.

Self-consciousness about the shape you are in. You may feel you are beyond the Speedo-limit, but the only way to get in shape is to get some exercise. You'll need to find a venue where you feel comfortable. A very young trainer looked at my birth year as though I were a time traveler; sometimes you need to keep your eye on the prize and let go of the rest.

Comparing yourself to others. Your pace, your program, your progress will all be yours alone. Share your celebrations with everyone.

Pessimism. Optimists confine an event to a day, pessimists make it universal. (*I missed my class, I'm blowing my program, I can never do it./ I missed my class, I'll be sure to make the next one.*)

Going for broke. Starting out at full throttle will tire your body, risk injury, and leave you dispirited. Start both your program and your individual sessions slowly and build up.

I have more important things to do. Speaking to myself when I (often) say that: Enough already.

Getting back on track

You may find life getting in the way of your exercise schedule with interruptions such as family obligations or travel. It happens in all of our lives. Just start again, but be careful about picking up where you left off if you have been increasing your program. Start at lesser intensity until you are comfortable, before you step it up.

Creative ways to exercise

Think of ways you can integrate more exercise into your daily life.

The average American spends, over a lifetime, an average of six months waiting at red lights. You can use the time by exercising your hands with a foam ball or doing an isometric scan of your body, tightening and relaxing muscle groups from your face to your feet.

While you are sitting on hold on the phone or watching television, roll a tennis ball or a rolling pin under your foot. Without a ball, inscribe words or loops in the air with your foot—a good flexibility exercise for traveling. Don't laugh. I've used this in a lecture to remind myself of what I have to pick up at the store on my way home.

Try the Amish program: Walk as much as possible in the normal course of your day. Take the stairs instead of the elevator, and park your car on the far side of the parking lot. Because they are not automated, the Amish walk about three times as much per day on average than we do and are significantly less overweight.

Get a pedometer to keep track of the number of steps you take during the day. A mile is two thousand to two thousand five hundred steps. Most working people average four thousand steps per day. An additional forty-five to sixty-minute walk will bring the total up to ten thousand. If you are a quantifier, it may help you stay with your program to have a record of how far you travel.

Lift weights while you watch the evening news. Or exercise your hands with a handgrip with handles that are squeezed together (they come in different resistances), with Chinese balls to rotate in the palm, or with squeeze balls.

Do range-of-motion exercises at your desk. Periodic shoulder or head rolls will reinvigorate you.

Ride your bike to local destinations—to the store, to a friend's house, to work.

Take a walk on your lunch break. Or take a walk with your dog or your stroller. If you don't have a baby, you'd be giving a gift to the parents, as well as yourself, to push the child of friends along on a walk.

Add a CD player or an iPod to your exercise session so that you can listen to music or recorded books. A good audio book can get you out to walk, and audio books are available from your library.

Electronic options

A substantial number of people choose to exercise without the supervision of a professional. A wide variety of exercise classes are offered on television. I have recorded a five A.M. yoga class to follow at a more convenient time. It worked for a while, but I found it impersonal and hard to stick with, and I discovered later, in a live class, that my form needed a great deal of correction.

Still, exercising at home with some guidance is the best option for some people. Home fitness videos and DVD's, some of which are sold by the Arthritis Foundation, are also available.

Online training programs are increasingly popular for those who want to exercise at home with accountability to a trainer. About 8 percent of trainers work online, and the trainers range from those who lack credentials to exercise physiologists. Most work with a questionnaire to create personal workouts, and clients can keep track of progress on the trainer's site, ask questions electronically, or call. For many, the accountability, even without personal contact, helps them stay with a program.

The gardening cure

My father-in-law, who has never been much for exercise programs, stays fit by spending hours gardening. Hoeing, digging, weeding, pruning, pushing a wheelbarrow, lifting debris, and planting can be good for maintaining joint flexibility, bone density, range of motion and quality of life. In his case, his routine exams have shown a remarkable improvement in his health. Researchers at the University of Arkansas found that active gardening ranks as high as weight training for strengthening bones.

As with any activity, be sure to consult your doctor or physical therapist for any precautions you should take. For example a brace can provide support for a sore joint.

Plan to work in the garden when you feel best, if you have morning stiffness or afternoon fatigue. Stretch before you start and begin with lighter work. Use tools with large handles or wrap them yourself with foam padding to avoid stress on your hands.

Keep your back straight and sit on an overturned bucket or gardening stool to plant. You might find raised beds helpful. Planting organic vegetables and flowers without the use of pesticides is a good choice, as environmental toxins can be causal for RA.

IN A SENTENCE:

> *Getting on course with an exercise program can take consideration of what gets in the way and creativity in choosing what you will stick with.*

FIRST-MONTH MILESTONE

Your learning curve over this month has been steep. It has lifted you up out of any doubt that you can manage your RA. You have learned that:

○ THE WAY YOU LOOK AT THE WORLD IS MAL-
LEABLE, AND IT CAN INFLUENCE THE OUT-
COME OF YOUR RA PROGRAM.

○ NEGATIVE SELF-TALK CAN BE REPLACED
WITH INTERNAL MESSAGES THAT WILL SUP-
PORT YOUR GOALS.

○ YOU CAN TRANSFORM STRESS INTO A HOPE
FILLED OUTLOOK, TO YOUR BENEFIT.

○ EXERCISE IS THE BEST NONPHARMA-
CEUTICAL MEDICINE FOR RA, AND THAT YOU
NEED A REGULAR PROGRAM WITH RANGE-OF-
MOTION, STRENGTH TRAINING, AND AEROBIC
COMPONENTS.

Keeping a Journal

Several journals can be helpful

Journals are useful tools for charting both progress and failures in order to establish a realistic basis for your next step. You can use journals for diverse purposes. You may find benefit from three kinds:

○ A *medical journal* to record symptoms, medications, supplements, test results, and notes for your doctor.
○ A *goals journal* divided into parts for exercise, nutrition, and other contributions to your well-being.
○ A *personal journal* to record your thoughts and feelings— a task with more purpose than may be evident at first glance.

I use regular loose-leaf binders, and some people like spiral notebooks. A nicely bound blank book is a pleasure to use for the personal journal, but any format will do. You can put all of the information in one binder, but bear in mind that you take your medical journal to appointments with your doctor, so you won't want it to be unwieldy. There are also preprinted journals for health, exercise, or diet, called the Memory Minder (see Resources), and many people, like my husband, prefer to store data on a computer.

Keeping medical records

There are many reasons for keeping a medical journal, and any one of them makes the effort worthwhile. You can keep track of your response to changes in your program—medication, exercise, relaxation practices. Also, a medical journal will shorten the information gathering part of your doctor's appointment, allowing more time in the visit for your questions. Although accumulating details may seem like a task, they form useful patterns that your doctor can read. You can use your journal to note questions for your appointment as they arise. Keep track, too, of routine but essential primary care.

You have a lot of joints, and it can be hard to remember which are affected, how much, when, and for how long. Keep track of your symptoms on a chart, weekly at first, while you are settling into a program, then monthly. You need to note them before your doctor's appointment or when you change part of your program, such as your medication, exercise regimen, or relaxation practice.

Beside your medical history, which you will need for your first visit, you need to chart your medications, including vitamins and supplements, with dosage, and how often taken.

Keeping track of joint pain and inflammation is often done using an established system for charting pain on a scale of zero to ten, from none to unbearable. You will need to be able to record which joints are involved and when. Note this information weekly at first, unless your RA is changing rapidly, in which case you might keep a semiweekly log for a while.

Fatigue, the body's reaction to substances released into the bloodstream by activated immune cells, is an indicator of your condition. Your records need to show its time and duration. Any other symptoms, such as low-grade fever, loss of appetite, depression, anemia, or the appearance of rheumatoid nodules, need to be noted.

Dryness of the eyes, mouth, or vagina can indicate RA-related Sjögren's syndrome, and need to be recorded for mention to the doctor.

Ask for copies of tests to be sent to you and to any other physician treating you. Add information to your journal from your visit to the doctor—test results, blood pressure, and what the doctor said.

I keep a page in the notebook to write questions as they come up between appointments. Some I can answer by looking them up in RA resources. When I am ready for the appointment, I choose the most important few that I have no answers for. At one time it was always about some wonder cure. Now it tends to be about something I have read or the long-term efficacy of a drug I am taking.

This journal is a logistical aid, but you will also use it for the pleasure of turning back in it to see how far you have come—a pleasure that can't help but tickle some beneficial neuron.

Recording primary care tests

It bears repeating that RA patients are less likely to keep up with routine medical care that requires a special appointment. Perhaps, with all of our doctor visits, enough is enough—an understandable feeling. We are, as a group, up until now anyway, statistically more prone to health complications beyond the immediate symptoms of RA, so it is more important for us than for many people to attend to primary care assessments.

The following charts list the recommendations of the American Academy of Family Physicians and the Centers for Disease Control (CDC). These are routine tests, listed by age, for people who are not at special risk for serious complications. If your family history or medication predisposes you to particular illnesses, you and your doctor need to discuss further testing.

Again, have the results of these tests sent both to your rheumatologist and to you to keep in your medical journal.

Use your goals journal every day

Even if you are a person who can keep a lot in your head, like phone numbers and birthdays, and who has never considered needing a notebook full of reminders, you will find that there is a lot more to reckon with now. Consider creating a goals journal if any part of your RA program is still under construction. It's a building plan, a map to guide you.

In each area, you can chart first your overall goal and then the portion of it you want to achieve in a week. It is important to set a time frame instead of floating along in an endless succession of tomorrows. The section in Day 3 on making a plan will take you through the process of breaking down your goals.

In some areas, I have not had to make notes for years. Others seem to be ongoing works in progress. For those, I like to look at the week on a single sheet, so I can see how I am doing. I also like to make a note of distractions or barriers so that patterns will become apparent. It's odd not to be aware, but in looking at my notes I realized I was skipping exercise on Monday mornings because I was sleeping late. I'd miss it on Wednesdays because I was preparing lunch for a weekly musical session my husband has with a dear friend. I had to choose between my exercise goal and sleeping or cooking. Monday was solved with the alarm clock, Wednesday by the Crock-Pot with a pot of soup made the night before. It seems simple in retrospect, but moving through it takes attention that can be nudged by a written goal.

Exercise journal

Exercise gives the most guaranteed short- and long-term relief to arthritis pain and stiffness. It will improve your overall strength, energy, balance, and coordination. It will improve your circulation as well as bone density and muscle flexibility. This is the no-brainer in the RA program.

You will need to incorporate three kinds of exercise: range-of-motion, strength training, and aerobic exercise. Each has a purpose, and each type will have a goal and a schedule for you to record. (See the exercise chapters in Weeks 3 and 4.)

If you are not already keeping track of your body mass index (BMI), and your heart rate when you do aerobic exercise, learn how to do both.

Nutrition journal

You may have established good nutritional habits like one svelte friend of mine who has been eating whole grains and organic vegetables for years—in which case you don't need to log your food. If you are more like me, you may need a program to help you become more careful about what and how much you eat. You have read, and it will bear repeating, that taking off ten pounds will take thirty pounds of stress off your joints. A new study makes that forty pounds.

Even if your weight is neatly under control, stay with me here, because the quality of your nutrition does influence your overall health. There is no "arthritis diet," no matter how many books by that title you may have seen or how many miracle food cures you may have heard about. Still, what you eat is so important that I suggest you chart it until you are satisfied that you have established good habits.

Don't bite off more than you can chew, so to speak; make your goals small. You can replace ice cream with yogurt, butter with olive oil, white bread with whole wheat, or white rice with brown. Just keep the small changes coming, and record your victories every week. Making note of what you eat will make you conscious, and, as with every element of change, awareness is the first step.

Journal for well-being

This is the section to use for various goals to reduce stress. Remember that the stress caused by RA is both physical and emotional. Included in the journal can be plans for pacing your activities; relaxation practices such as meditation, visualization, yoga, or tai chi. If you tend to isolate yourself and need to make an effort to stay socially connected, you may want to make that a goal. This journal can also contain notes on your mood or barriers to success.

Sleep and rest log

You may find that lying down once or twice a day will help your fatigue, but it is difficult to incorporate into your routine. This or any other element of your program that you are introducing will benefit from getting a goal page of its own, to be monitored weekly until the practice is adopted. For most people, once they do integrate rest regularly into a broader program, the need to monitor it eventually diminishes.

If sleep is a problem, it may help to make notes on elements of your progress.

Log for simplifying and organizing

Simplifying and organizing are ongoing objectives for me. I find it helpful to focus on a single project; otherwise, nothing gets done. There is wide latitude in this section, according to your choice and according to the areas in your program that require structure. You may choose to add your personal journal to this section rather than use a separate book.

Resources

Add a running list of resources at the back—contact information for members of your team, class and support group schedules, notes on Web sites or books to read. In the pocket in the back of your notebook or in an envelope, save relevant articles to discuss in your support group or with your doctor.

Take a dose of journal

A study similar to those done with the gratitude journals described in the last chapter involved RA patients writing about life experience. Those taking part were directed to write about their "deepest thoughts and feelings" continuously for twenty minutes. The results, published in the *Journal of the American Medical Association*, concluded that the experience had a positive influence on the health of a significant number of the participants.

Writing about events in our lives allows us to externalize them and reconsider the way we think about them. The restructuring of perception, called narrative repair by psychologists, can reduce levels of stress and bring about physical benefits. You may find that keeping your personal journal next to your bed will remind you to write, if not every night, then often.

Okay, so maybe you don't think of yourself as the heart-on-the-page kind of person. Fair enough. There are no course requirements here. Keep in mind, though, that getting well is not one-stop shopping. Every little act contributes. Journal writing is therapeutic and the price is right. But fishing is free, and that may serve you, too.

IN A SENTENCE:

> *Keeping journals provides both practical records and a valuable means of reviewing and restructuring experience.*

learning

Journal Pages

THE FOLLOWING record-keeping pages will help you organize your journal. Keeping your medical information in order is crucial to your care. Other areas, in which you are creating change, will benefit from systematic notes. Refer back to Month 2, Living for a discussion on how to keep each one of these journal pages. You may choose to copy and use these, a commercial form mentioned in the Resources section, or a system of your own devising that will grow out of these pages.

Weekly Medical Journal

Dates: _____ to _____, 20___ weight _____

SYMPTOMS

Joint pain and stiffness (rated 1–10)	Left	Right
Neck		
Shoulders		
Elbows		
Wrists		
Thumb base		
1st joint		
Finger 1 knuckle		
1st joint		
Finger 2 knuckle		
1st joint		
Finger 3 knuckle		
1st joint		
Finger 4 knuckle		
1st joint		
Hips		
Knees		
Ankles		
Feet		

Duration of morning stiffness:

Means of relief:

Dryness: ○ Mouth ○ Eyes

Other symptoms:

Fatigue: Time of day, duration:

Means of relief:

Medications, vitamins, herbs, supplements / dosage / frequency:

Notes on how you feel in general:

Primary care

The following are routine tests recommended by the American Academy of Family Physicians and the Centers for Disease Control (CDC), listed by age.

FIVE-YEAR PRIMARY CARE TESTING CHART AGES 19–39

Test/Frequency	Year of test				
	20__	20__	20__	20__	20__
Blood pressure Annually					
Blood glucose Annually after age 25					
Cancer checkup to detect cancer of the thyroid, mouth, skin, and lymph nodes, plus testes and prostate for men and ovaries for women. Every 3 years after age 20					
Cholesterol test Every 5 years					
Glaucoma Every 2–3 years starting at age 35					
Syphilis and gonorrhea Annually or more frequently, depending on number of sexual partners					
Breast exam (women) Doctor's exam every 3 years after age 20. Self-exam every month.					
Mammogram (women) Once between ages 35 and 39					
Pap test/pelvic exam (women) Annually or at doctor's discretion					

FIVE-YEAR PRIMARY CARE TESTING CHART AGES 40-49

Test/Frequency	Year of test				
	20__	20__	20__	20__	20__
Blood pressure, vision, hearing, blood glucose, blood count, cancer and urine analysis for sugar and protein Annually					
Digital rectal exam Annually					
Cancer checkup to detect cancer of the thyroid, mouth, skin, and lymph nodes, plus testes and prostate for men and ovaries for women. Every 3 years					
Cholesterol test Every 5 years					
Glaucoma Every 2–3 years					
Electrocardiogram Once between ages 40 and 45, then every 3–5 years					
Breast exam (women) Doctor's exam annually. Self-exam every month.					
Mammogram (women) Every 1–2 years					
Pap test/pelvic exam (women) Annually					

FIVE-YEAR PRIMARY CARE TESTING CHART AGES 50-64

Test/Frequency	Year of test				
	20__	20__	20__	20__	20__
Blood pressure, vision, hearing, blood glucose, blood count, cancer and urine analysis for sugar and protein Annually					
Cancer checkup to detect cancer of the thyroid, mouth, skin, and lymph nodes, plus testes and prostate for men and ovaries for women. Every 3 years					
Cholesterol test Every 5 years					
Digital rectal exam Annually					
Electrocardiogram Every 3–5 years					
Glaucoma Every 2–3 years					
Stool blood test Annually					
Sigmoidoscopy At age 50 and again at 51, then every 3–5 years					
Proctological exam (men) At age 50, again at 51, then every 3–5 years					
Breast exam (women) Doctor's exam annually. Self-exam every month.					
Mammogram (women) Annually					
Pap test/pelvic exam (women) Annually					

FIVE-YEAR PRIMARY CARE TESTING CHART AGES 65 AND OVER

Test/Frequency	Year of test					
	20__	20__	20__	20__	20__	20__
Cancer checkup to detect cancer of the thyroid, mouth, skin, and lymph nodes, plus testes and prostate for men and ovaries for women. Every 3 years						
Cholesterol test Every 5 years						
Digital rectal exam Annually						
Electrocardiogram Every 3–5 years						
Flu shots, blood pressure, vision, hearing, blood glucose, blood count, cancer, and urine analysis for sugar and protein Annually						
Glaucoma Every 2–3 years						
Sigmoidoscopy At age 50 and again at 51, then every 3–5 years						
Stool blood test Annually						
Proctological exam (men) Every 3–5 years						
Breast exam (women) Doctor's exam annually. Self-exam every month.						
Mammogram (women) Annually						
Pap test/pelvic exam (women) Annually						

Weekly Exercise Journal

Dates: _____ to _____, 20 _____

weight: _____

BMI: _____

WEEKLY GOALS

Range-of-motion exercise

Frequency: _____ × per week.

Duration: _____ minutes per session.   Time of day: _____

Description: _____

_____

Strength training

Frequency: _____ × per week.

Duration: _____ minutes per session.   Time of day: _____

Description: _____

_____

Aerobic exercise

Frequency: _____ × per week.

Duration: _____ minutes per session.   Time of day: _____

Starting heart rate: _____   Maximum heart rate: _____ for _____ minutes

Description: _____

_____

GOALS MET

	Sunday	Monday	Tuesday	Wednesday	Thursday	Friday	Saturday
Range-of-motion							
Strength training							
Aerobic exercise							

Distractions or barriers: _____

_____

_____

Solutions: _____

_____

_____

Weekly Journal of Well-Being

Dates: _____ to _____, 20___   weight: _____

WEEKLY GOALS:

Relaxation practices (Meditation, yoga, tai chi, prayer, massage, visualization, etc.)

Frequency: ____ × per week.   Duration: ____ minutes per session.   Time of day: _____

Description: _____

Goal met: _____

Pacing

Frequency: ____ × per week.   Duration: ____ minutes per session.   Time of day: _____

Description: _____

Goal met: _____

Social contacts

Frequency: ____ × per week.

Description: _____

Goal met: _____

Distractions or barriers: _____

Solutions: _____

Weekly Rest and Sleep Log

Dates: _____ to _____, 20___   weight: _____

REST

Goal: Frequency: ____ x per week.   Duration: ____ minutes per session.   Time of day: _____

Description: _____

Barriers to resting: _____

Solutions: _____

Goal met: _____

SLEEP

Goal: _____ hours of sleep per night.

	Sunday	Monday	Tuesday	Wednesday	Thursday	Friday	Saturday
Hours							

Day	Quality of sleep	Changes to improve sleep
Sunday		
Monday		
Tuesday		
Wednesday		
Thursday		
Friday		
Saturday		

Weekly Log for Simplifying and Organizing

Dates: _____ to _____, 20____

WEEKLY GOALS: to simplify and organize in small increments in the most frequented spaces.

At work

Frequency: _____ × per week.   Duration: _____ minutes per session.   Day/time: _____

Description: _____

_____

At home

Frequency: _____ × per week.   Duration: _____ minutes per session.   Day/time: _____

Description: _____

_____

In the garage or garden

Frequency: _____ × per week.   Duration: _____ minutes per session.   Day/time: _____

Description: _____

_____

GOALS MET

Sunday	Monday	Tuesday	Wednesday	Thursday	Friday	Saturday

Distractions or barriers: _____

_____

_____

_____

_____

_____

Solutions: _____

_____

_____

_____

_____

Weekly Nutrition Journal

Dates: _____ to _____, 20___   weight: _____

Goal	Nutrition	Sunday	Monday	Tuesday	Wednesday	Thursday	Friday	Saturday
8 glasses	water (juice, non-caffeinated drink)							
3 servings	vegetables							
3 servings	fruit							
4–9 servings	whole grain if possible; bread, cereal, rice, pasta							
1 serving	fish, soy, nuts, legumes							
2 servings	meat, poultry, eggs							
2 servings	milk, yogurt, cheese							
carefully	fats and oils rich in omega-3 fatty acids							
minimally	sweets							
daily	multi-vitamin							

Distractions or barriers to success:

Solutions:

living

Nutrition and RA

Common sense and the RA diet

The seduction of a food cure calls through the Internet, from the shelves of the bookstore, in the casual conversation of a well-meaning friend. It goes: So-and-so, often followed by initials of some sort, was a successful such-and-such until his work was cut short by crippling arthritis. Against all odds he fought back, gave up on prescribed medications, and devised a miracle diet that has cured him completely—along with scores of others.

As much as I wish I could chew my way out of this disease, there is no proven diet cure for RA. At the same time, there is no doubt that what you eat affects your immune system, and you can modify your nutrition to greatly benefit your condition.

It is true that there are people with food allergies that can worsen RA symptoms, but only one of the one hundred types of arthritis—gout—has been linked to what you eat.

So many painstakingly added links in an interdependent chain need to be assembled in a good RA program, and each is varied and uncertain; it's hard to tell when relief comes from a remedy or the natural flux of the disease. It's all too easy to become frustrated and reach for a quick fix.

How do you sort out fact from fiction?

The scapegoat diets

Superstition surrounded the tomato, thought to be poisonous when it came to Europe from the New World; a last outpost of such folk beliefs is in remedies for diseases without clear cures. Here is a sampler of the unproven diets that shun groups of foods as the causes of arthritis:

Nightshade vegetables. One of the most common diet claims is that eliminating nightshades relieves arthritis. These include tomatoes, potatoes, eggplants, and most peppers. There is no evidence that this is
true.

The alkaline diet. This diet assumes that OA and RA are caused by too
much acid. The diet excludes sugar, coffee, red meat, most grains,
nuts, and citrus fruit—eliminating most vitamin C sources. Apart from
the fact that the two diseases are related only by symptom, there is no
supporting evidence for this theory.

The Dong diet. This especially restrictive diet eliminates tomatoes, fruits,
red meat, herbs, dairy products, and alcohol. There's no evidence it
has a positive effect on arthritis.

Cleansing diets, fasting. Treatments are promoted as cleansing the body
of toxins to allow the body's natural curative powers to cure disease.
Accounts of improvement in RA during fasting may be related to a
temporary impairment of the immune system, but no sustained benefit has been found. Be cautious about fasting at a time when exercise and good nutrition are important.

Other such diets blame flour, bran, honey, cocoa, tea, salt, pepper, vinegar, and chocolate. None of these diets has been shown to be helpful, and
some may result in deficiencies of beneficial nutrients. Before you eliminate
a food group, check with your doctor.

The influence of diet on RA

Several studies have shown connections between diet and RA. The team headed by Dr. Lindsey Criswell, who does rheumatoid arthritis genet-ics research at the University of California at San Francisco, examined a body of data gathered over eleven years from half of the middle-aged women in the state in the Iowa (**The Iowa Women's Health Study**). It was possible to examine 40,000 dietary assessments, and to compare those of people who were eventually diagnosed with RA. Once again, your mother was right; eat your spinach. It appears that antioxidants have a positive effect against the development or progression of RA—particularly vitamins C, E, and A. Benefit was found in diets high in fruits and cruciferous vegetables. Citrus fruits, particularly oranges, were cited. Among cruciferous vegetables (cabbage, cauliflower), broccoli showed the strongest benefit—one of the few protective factors for RA.

Other studies have shown RA joints to have an excess of free oxygen radicals, by-products of the normal activity of cells that are believed to contribute to joint damage. The level of vitamin C in the joint fluid and blood of people with RA has been shown to be lower than normal. These facts support the Iowa study supposition that antioxidant vitamins and minerals could help protect cells against damage from free radicals.

There was enough suggestive evidence in the Iowa study to generate the hypothesis that vitamin D may reduce the risk of an immunologic disorder. Vitamin D and calcium in skim milk appeared to have a positive effect. It is known that vitamin D has immunologic activity, and in animal models it has been shown to be an immunosuppressant. Within the joint, locally produced vitamin D may help to decrease inappropriate T cell proliferation (see Month 7 for an explanation of the way the immune system works in RA).

Studies at Tufts University have shown that people with RA have an increased need for vitamins B6 (found in bananas, poultry, fish, beef) and folate (also a B vitamin, found in green leafy vegetables, citrus, grains). It is theorized that the need for these vitamins is created by inflammation.

The influence of medications

Some medications can produce nutritional deficits, for example steroids, which cause the body to lose potassium and retain sodium, or methotrexate, which requires supplementary folate. Some drugs cause gastrointestinal upset, like NSAIDs, that could interfere with the absorption of nutrients.

Weighing in

In Tudor England, it took hundreds of farmers, hunters, butchers, and cooks to keep Henry VIII fat. In America today, no one needs any help putting on weight by eating cheap fast food and abundant fatty, sugary snacks. The anthropologist George Armelagos observes that it takes an equivalent support team to keep Oprah from looking like Henry VIII—a personal trainer, a nutritionist, and a private chef. For those of us who have to do it on our own, it seems like such a formidable task to keep weight in check that many check out. The government reports that 65 percent of adults ages twenty to seventy-four are overweight, and nearly half of this group is obese.

The stakes are too high with RA not to control weight. Every extra pound adds stress on the knees—further compromising joints that are already affected by the disease. Losing ten pounds can cut the risk of damage by as much as half. Tendons and ligaments, which can be weakened by RA, can become separated by layers of fat, making them susceptible to bursitis and tendinitis.

Fat cells, until recently thought to be simple stores of excess energy, have been shown to produce and regulate many metabolic and hormonal signals that can affect the endocrine system. Fat tissue attracts immune system cells, macrophages (see Month 7), which promote inflammation. Dr. Gokhan Hotamisligil, Professor of Genetics and Metabolism at the Harvard School of Public Health, says, "If you have excess fat, even in small amounts, the body starts mounting an immune response, almost as if the body is perceiving excess calories as an invading organism." Cris Slentz, an exercise physiologist at Duke University, adds, "Fat cells put out cytokines . . . They increase inflammation." The role of this phenomenon in RA is not yet clear, but there is reason enough to keep excess weight off joints.

The myth of inevitability

The assumption that weight gain is a consequence of aging, particularly for women at menopause, is based on observation. What is not visible are the missed opportunities for staying fit. It has been shown that the imbalance causing weight gain in menopausal women is not hormonal but calories in versus calories out. As many ways as I have tried to cheat the laws of physics, it comes down to exercise and nutrition to keep fit. There is no way around it; both are necessary for controlling weight. Diets don't work. The best plan is a gradual lifestyle change.

Sleep is another influence on weight control. Chronic lack of sleep has been shown to cause a hormone that increases appetite to rise and one that suppresses appetite to fall substantially. Dr. Eve Van Cuter of the University of Chicago concludes that "if you are sleep-deprived, you will crave high-carb foods."

The new food pyramid

The USDA Dietary Guidelines for Americans 2005, the latest version of the familiar food pyramid, recommends that you:

1. Consume fewer calories. Eat more fruits, vegetables, and whole grains and less meat, dairy, sugar, fat, and foods high in simple carbohydrates. Avoid trans fats (margarine, vegetable shortening, partially hydrogenated oils).
2. Exercise more (to maintain weight, an hour a day, to lose weight, an hour and a half). The new graphic symbol is a triangular chart with a runner ascending stairs up the side of the triangle to show the

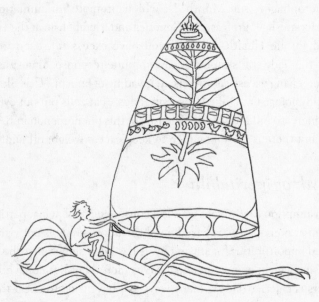

The nutritional needs of RA are answered by a healthy diet. From the bottom: water, the base, transports nutrients; fruits and vegatables; fish, meat, beans; dairy products; whole grains; polyunsaturated fats; recreational foods such as sugar.

importance of exercise. At Mypyramid.gov you can key in your age, sex, and current amount of exercise to get recommended daily amounts for each food group.

The *New York Times* estimates that only 2 to 4 percent of people eat according to the guidelines, so they might be more usefully considered to be an ideal than an impossibility.

Cutting density

If you have dieted, you know the feeling of being hungry and deprived. Chances are that whatever weight you lost is back on board. In fact, studies have shown that the way for thin people to gain weight is to go on a diet; the metabolism is slowed and the body creates extra stores.

It has been found that people tend to eat the same volume of food every day, so the trick to keeping weight down is to eat foods that are higher in volume and lower in calories. Water adds the greatest volume to most foods, so water-rich foods, like vegetables, fruits, and broth-based soups are good choices. Researchers at Pennsylvania State University have found that three elements of food produce satiety—low-calorie density, high fiber, and lean protein. It is a nice coincidence that foods with these qualities can handsomely supply our nutritional needs.

Talking to the food is a strategy suggested by Dr. Beth Tabakin, who specializes in weight problems. Rather than entertaining the feeling that you can't have something because you are too heavy, "look at the food and say 'Are you good enough for my fine body?'" Another of Dr. Tabakin's mental exercises is to imagine the coveted food as your mate in life. Chocolate cake, she concludes, "looks good, smells good, is great in bed—and you feel abused after each night together . . . It's like being with a beautiful man who treats me badly." These kinds of things can seem dippy, but there is method to the madness. It is a process of becoming conscious, and you might want to invent your own script.

Laugh it off

If you're up for a comedy, spontaneous laughter increases your calorie requirement by 20 percent, according to a study at Vanderbilt University.

Sorry, forced laughter is regulated by a separate part of the brain; it has to be the real thing. Half an hour of guffawing will get you an ounce of chocolate, so it had better be a funny show.

Guidelines for a healthy arthritis diet

You have a lot to manage with RA, and controlling your fuel resources will control a lot of other parts of your program. The Arthritis Foundation's nutritional guidelines include familiar recommendations: eat a variety of foods (you need over forty essential nutrients); maintain optimum weight; include enough starch and fiber; avoid excess fat, cholesterol, sugar, and salt; consume alcohol in moderation.

Add to that water, the physiologic river upon which nutrients navigate the body. The eight-glass rule is debatable, but drink water rather than caffeinated drinks or alcohol because they are diuretics.

In place of processed foods, choose what looks as close as possible to the same when you eat it as it did when it was picked.

Fruits and vegetables. **Antioxidants** that may help reduce inflammation are found in fruits and vegetables. The Iowa study particularly cites the benefits of antioxidants in oranges and broccoli. The USDA ranks the top ten foods containing antioxidants as: blueberries, kale, strawberries, spinach, Brussels sprouts, plums, broccoli, beets, oranges, red grapes. (Dark chocolate has more antioxidants than blueberries.)

The government food pyramid has increased the recommended intake of fruits and vegetables from five to nine servings a day; it seems like a lot until you consider that the servings, a miniscule half cup reminiscent of an elementary school cafeteria, total four and a half cups. It's quite doable: Start with morning orange juice, a piece of fruit for midmorning snack, salad with lunch, an afternoon smoothie, vegetable with dinner, and fruit for dessert. Aim to vary vegetable subgroups throughout the week—dark green, orange, legumes (beans and peas), starchy vegetables, and others. The cruciferous vegetables, identified as beneficial by the Iowa study, include: cabbage, broccoli, Brussels sprouts, beet greens, cauliflower, kale, parsley, Swiss chard. Rule of thumb: go for color.

Meat, poultry, fish, eggs, and beans. You can boost your intake of omega-3, thought to reduce inflammation, by choosing more vegetable proteins—tofu, beans, nuts, and seeds. This shift to plant-based proteins along with fish and less meat, dubbed the flexitarian diet, is becoming more common. Eggs have had a bad rap because the yolks contain some cholesterol, but researchers at Harvard have concluded that an egg a day is a healthy source of protein, vitamins B_{12} and D, riboflavin, and folate—a good package for the RA diet. Choose leaner cuts of meat and forget the chicken skin.

Dairy products are an important source of calcium, crucial for the health of bones in RA. Surveys have shown that many people do not consume adequate amounts. Animal experiments suggest a possible benefit from yogurt for RA. Choose low-fat products.

Grains. The importance placed by the USDA and the Arthritis Foundation on grains counters the claims of low-carbohydrate diets, which seem to be at the end of the fad cycle anyway. Choose whole grains most often.

Salt and additives. Aim to consume less than a teaspoon of salt (2,300 mg) per day, using other spices to flavor food. Read labels; there is a lot of salt in packaged foods.

Fats. Out with the bad: trans fats (mostly found in fast foods, commercial baking, shortening, margarine) and saturated fats (mainly animal fats in whole milk, butter, cheese, red meat, but some are found in plant foods such as coconut oil, palm kernel oil).

Out with the almost as bad: polyunsaturated fats (corn, soybean, safflower, cottonseed oils).

In with the good: monounsaturated fats (olive oil, canola oil, peanut oil, cashews, almonds, peanuts, most other nuts, avocados).

The general health benefits of this change make it worthwhile; in addition, there is evidence that the switch can have a positive affect on inflammation in RA.

Oiling your joints

Oils contain fatty acids that make their way to the membranes of the cells, including the cells in joints. It has been observed that some fatty acids, called omega-6, appear to fuel inflammation; they are found in meats as well as oils such as cottonseed and corn. Others, omega-3 fatty acids, appear to decrease inflammation; they are polyunsaturated, like the fats in plants, and are found in cold-water fish, free-range eggs, and flax seeds.

It was discovered that peoples whose diets were based on deep sea fish, such as the Inuit of Greenland, get less arthritis (but the study does not compare Inuit on Western diets). Possible benefit to RA inspired several studies using high doses of fish oil. Subjects reported a reduction in joint tenderness and morning stiffness, but the high dosages also produced belching, gas, and fishy breath. Fish oil also thins the blood. In a Danish study more close to normal intake, RA patients ate four ounces of fish every day and experienced a decrease in swelling and pain.

Find omega-3 in cold-water fish such as salmon, sardines, mackerel, trout, herring, sablefish, and sturgeon. You can find fish that are abundant, toxin free, or responsibly farmed at the Web site Monterey Bay Aquarium Seafood Watch (www.mbayaq.org and click seafood watch).

Vegetarian diet

The evidence is not clear, but there may be a positive relationship between RA and vegetarian diet. A small study showed improvement in four weeks, and follow-up studies of those who stayed on the diet showed continued improvement after one and two years. Other patterns have been shown by the research—for example, in one study overeating appeared to aggravate RA, and in another, vegans (who eat no dairy or animal products) reported less pain than meat eaters. Finnish researchers found that a diet of raw fruits and vegetables supplemented with lactobacillus—bacteria found in yogurt—appeared to be helpful for the half of RA patients that did not need to drop out of the study due to gastrointestinal upset. Animal experiments tend to support the theory that lactobacillus may be helpful to the immune system, at least in mice with RA.

If you do choose to eliminate meat from your diet, be sure to replace it with fish or vegetable proteins.

Protein requirement and rheumatoid cachexia

It has been shown that people with RA do not require supplementary protein, as was once theorized. A metabolic change found in rheumatoid arthritis patients, called **rheumatoid cachexia**, creates a loss of muscle, resulting in a lower than normal body cell mass (BCM). It was thought that this breakdown of protein in the body required a diet high in protein to supplement the loss. A study done under the auspices of the U.S. Department of Agriculture Human Nutrition Research Center on Aging has determined that the condition is a result of lower levels of exercise. The remedy is to get up, not to chow down.

Elimination diets

Very few people have a true food allergy that aggravates RA. The problem, of course, is that the disease comes and goes, so it is very difficult to know the cause of improvement. Nevertheless, you may want to try an elimination diet if you suspect you are hypersensitive to a food.

Stop eating the suspected food group (nuts, dairy) for a week or so before you add it back and see what happens. Follow the process several times to see if there is a change in your condition when you bring the food back into your diet. Some researchers suggest a minimum of six weeks for each food to see results. Be sure to get the missing nutrients from other foods.

Keep your food journal carefully along with your records of arthritis symptoms. You may see a pattern. Then again, you may not.

Alcohol and medications

Alcoholic beverages do have a high caloric content and can account for extra weight. Also, alcohol can interfere with the effectiveness of some arthritis drugs. Alcohol is contraindicated with methotrexate, although a rheumatologist told me that it is all right in conservative amounts. With NSAIDs, which include aspirin, you may be more likely to have stomach problems. Acetaminophen combined with large amounts of alcohol can cause liver damage. That being said, it seems that alcohol in moderation does not exacerbate RA, and you might find a glass of wine enjoyable from time to time.

> In the year 2090, results of an 85-year $75 billion study are reported: Exercise and eating right are the keys to good health.
>
> —INTERNET JOKE

IN A SENTENCE:

Although there is no proven arthritis diet, healthy eating habits are beneficial to RA.

Take Your Vitamins

Nutritional necessity

As this book has progressed, I have told you what I have learned and encouraged you to take from it what you choose. But now we come to necessity, not option. How can I tell you how important it is? I can say, "Eat well," but the words are lighter than the satisfaction of a juicy burger slathered with cheese on a fluffy white bun with a side of fries and a shake. The majority of Americans who regularly eat poorly risk a list of physical problems, ending all too often with the heart. Those of us with RA face the same hellish list and then some.

How can I tell you to mind your peas and cucumbers? When I was diagnosed, I needed to convince myself, someone who loved a deep-fried frosted doughnut. The truth is that there is nothing that tastes better than your right weight feels. So here are the vitamins and minerals that make you function, together with the deficiencies that can be found in active RA and the foods that replenish them. The moral is: if you want these body parts to work, eat this stuff.

Vitamins

The bad news is that RA, as well as other autoimmune diseases, often brings vitamin and mineral deficiencies—as a result rather than a cause. The good news is that good food and a daily multivitamin go a long way toward making them up.

What we know is that the body cannot make vitamins and that the best source of nutrients is a diet rich in fruits, vegetables, and whole grains. In addition to vitamins, there are more than 20 minerals in a balanced diet; they help regulate fluid balance, muscle contractions, and nerve impulses, and are critical for the development of bones and teeth.

Animal research has shown that vitamins A, B, C, D, and E are involved with the immune system, as are iron, zinc, copper, magnesium, and selenium. More is not necessarily better, though. Some vitamins, such as C, are water-soluble and the excess is excreted. Fat-soluble vitamins, like E, are stored in the tissue and can build up to toxic levels. Some supplements interfere with medications, and studies have come to conflicting conclusions as to benefits to RA symptoms, so it is wise to review your program with your doctor.

Alphabet soup: what the letters mean

The old RDA (**Recommended Dietary Allowances**) reference for food ingredients has been replaced by a system called **DVs (Daily Values)**. DVs comprise two sets of reference values for nutrients, consolidated to simplify.

The RDA was a system designed to prevent nutritional deficiencies. The DV is based on values created with the goal of decreasing the risk of chronic diseases through nutrition. You will see DV on labels to describe the amount of a nutrient based on a 2,000-calorie diet.

Apart from the addition of fluoride, the greatest difference is in an emphasis on calcium from dairy products, which studies show is often not consumed at recommended levels. The report also underlines the advantage of getting nutrients from food rather than from supplements because food provides components for which values are not yet determined.

Antioxidants

A popularly held theory that antioxidants can prevent cancer and heart disease has not proven to be true in numerous clinical trials. It has been thought that antioxidants can neutralize certain oxygen-reactive molecules, called free radicals, that contribute to disease and tissue damage. But antioxidants may work through different pathways. Whether star or understudy, antioxidant-rich foods are associated with positive effects in RA.

A vitamin primer

Vitamin A (beta-carotene or retinoids). Beta-carotene, the plant-derived precursor to this fat-soluble vitamin, has the advantage of very low toxicity and is a superior antioxidant. Vitamin A is required for normal immune system function, protects eyesight, and keeps skin and tissues healthy. Although low levels are found in people with RA, no studies have shown that a supplement benefits the disease. High levels of A from retinol have been shown to raise the risk of bone fracture; beta-carotene does not appear to have this effect. Take no more than 100 percent daily value (DV) of retinol and beta-carotene combined. Because it is a fat-soluble vitamin, A is toxic in high doses; it is best to get it from the diet.

Foods containing beta-carotene: apricots, cantaloupe, carrots, dark leafy greens, mango. Foods containing retinol: beef, chicken, fish, eggs, fortified milk.

Vitamin B. This vitamin comprises several water-soluble vitamins, each functioning separately in widely differing roles. When these vitamins were discovered nearly a hundred years ago, it was mistakenly believed that there was only one vitamin B, hence one name for them all. Studies have shown that some people with arthritis are deficient in B vitamins. Among the reasons: several arthritis drugs, including aspirin, can deplete the body of B vitamins. Also, patients were found to consume far fewer foods rich in B than they needed.

Foods containing B vitamins: whole grains, fish, green leafy vegetables.

B_1, *Thiamine.* B_1 converts sugar to energy and is essential for the normal functioning of the heart, brain, nervous system, and muscles.

Absorption is decreased with excessive amounts of coffee, tea, or alcohol, as well as oral contraceptives, antibiotics, sulfa drugs, regular use of antacids, and some diuretics. Most supplements provide 100 percent of the DV.

Foods containing B_1: Fish, pork, sunflower seeds, whole wheat, brown rice, lentils, peas, beans. Foods fortified with thiamine include pasta, bread, rice, and cereal.

B_2, *riboflavin*. B_2 aids in the generation of skin and red blood cells and helps convert sugar to energy. It is usually contained in B complex vitamin pills; B_2 is unstable in light.

Foods containing B_2: beef, milk, cheese, eggs, almonds, fortified cereals, and grains.

B_3, *niacin*. B_3 helps transform sugars and fats into energy, and helps maintain tissue of the skin and the digestive system. Doses over the DV can cause nausea and headache, and high doses can cause ulcers or liver damage.

Foods containing B_3: chicken, tuna, turkey, fish, beef, peanut butter.

B_5, *pantothenic acid*. In an early study people with RA were shown to be deficient in B_5. Another small study showed some reduction in symptoms with a supplement.

Food containing B_5: soybeans, lentils, eggs, grains, meat.

B_6, *pyridoxine*. B_6 is required for the formation of red blood cells and antibodies and is important for nerve and brain function as well as energy production—among one hundred chemical reactions in the body. Inflammation in RA may decrease the level of B_6, according to an Arthritis Foundation funded study at Tufts University. In taking a supplement, do not exceed 100 percent of the DV. Long-term high doses can lead to nerve damage.

Foods containing B_6: bananas, salmon, beans, potatoes, chicken, peanut butter.

B_{12}, *cobalamin*. B_{12} helps make red blood cells, nerve cells, and genetic material and converts folate to its active form. Anemia, caused by folate deficiency, can be a problem in RA, so adequate B_{12} is crucial, particularly when taking methotrexate. Supplements are advised for vegetarians and people over fifty because B_{12} absorption declines with age.

Foods containing B_{12}: meat, poultry, fish, eggs, dairy product, leafy green vegetables, legumes, peanuts, sunflower seeds, whole grains.

Vitamin C, ascorbic acid. Vitamin C builds and maintains collagen and connective tissue, helps form red blood cells, aids the absorption of iron and folic acid, and expedites wound healing. In its role as an antioxidant, it may be beneficial to inflammation in RA. It is thought to bind free radicals, which can damage cartilage and cause swelling. Although findings for OA do not necessarily translate to RA, it is worth noting that osteoarthritis patients with the most antioxidants in their diets had significantly lower chances of progressive damage. Further damage was reduced by two-thirds in those with OA who had a high vitamin C level.

Bruising that sometimes comes with RA has been known to improve with 500 milligrams a day of this water-soluble vitamin, and it may also improve the effectiveness of aspirin. It is thought that natural and synthetic C have the same effect. Added ingredients such as rose hips or bioflavonoids have not been shown to be beneficial. NSAIDs, antibiotics, and steroids increase the need for C.

Foods containing C: citrus fruits, melons, green leafy vegetables, tomatoes, peppers, pineapple, strawberries, papaya, broccoli, Brussels sprouts, kiwi.

Vitamin D. This is a fat-soluble vitamin that is essential for building and maintaining teeth and bones. It aids in the absorption of calcium and phosphorus. It comes mostly through exposure to the sun, although it is found in food as well. In a study of osteoarthritis of the knee, researchers found that patients with a diet high in D, or taking a supplement, experienced a significant reduction in joint damage.

Steroids can cause bone deterioration, and patients taking them are cautioned to include D-rich foods or supplements at no more than the DV, because all fat-soluble vitamins can be toxic in high doses.

Foods containing D: cold-water fish (such as salmon, sardines, mackerel, herring, tuna, anchovy, lake trout), dairy products, including fortified milk, egg yolks.

Vitamin E. This vitamin is arguably the most important antioxidant in the body, as it works to bind free radicals. It is essential to the formation of red blood cells and the maintenance of a normal immune system.

Low levels of vitamin E have been found in the inflamed joints of RA patients. Several studies have shown that people with RA do not consume enough E. Supplements have been reported in preliminary studies to be helpful, but high doses can interfere with blood clotting. E can interact with blood-thinning medications, aspirin, and NSAIDs.

Foods containing E: whole grains, nuts, poultry, fish, sunflower seeds, wheat germ, legumes, peanut butter, almonds, soybean oil, turnip greens.

Folate, folic acid. Folate is active in red blood cell development, cell reproduction, and the formation of DNA. It helps lower levels of homocysteine, linked to heart disease; a study at Tufts found people with RA to have increased levels of homocysteine.

Folic acid is a required supplement for people who take methotrexate. Most multivitamins include folic acid. It is recommended that half the intake should come from food.

Foods containing folic acid: leafy green vegetables (spinach, kale, collards, turnip greens), legumes, broccoli, dried beans, asparagus, black-eyed peas, lentils, peas, oranges, brown rice, whole grain breads and cereals.

Vitamin K. K promotes blood clotting and building of bones. Studies show that K levels are associated with bone mineral density; adequate K reduces the risk of fracture. K has only recently been added to some multivitamin formulas, but in amounts lower than the RDA because K can thin the blood.

Foods containing K: dark leafy greens, broccoli, Brussels sprouts, cabbage.

Minerals

Calcium. Calcium-rich bones are less susceptible to damage—a risk in RA. Some drugs taken for RA can reduce calcium levels in addition to the decline that comes with aging. Supplements can help, but they shouldn't replace foods high in calcium.

Foods containing calcium: low-fat milk, yogurt, calcium-fortified juice, tofu (with calcium sulfate), cheese, fish canned with bones such as sardines, salmon, and mackerel.

Chromium. This mineral helps the body process insulin, protein, fat, and carbohydrates. A supplement is not recommended.

Foods containing chromium: whole grains, wheat germ, brewer's yeast, green beans, prunes, nuts, peanut butter, potatoes, peas, eggs, cheese.

Copper. Although copper is found on most lists of bogus RA cures, a belief in its efficacy persists. According to the ancient Greeks, it has healing power, and traces of copper from bracelets worn by moderns subscribing to this belief are absorbed into the body. However, people with RA often have higher than average levels of copper in their blood, not lower. Although copper has been found to have anti-inflammatory properties, there has been no finding to support its use as an arthritis treatment. Copper does have a role in building red blood cells and connective tissue, as well as transporting iron.

Foods containing copper: oysters, crab, barley, beans, cashews, sunflower seeds, semisweet chocolate, peanut butter, lentils, mushrooms.

Fluoride. This mineral helps strengthen teeth and bones but cannot decrease bone loss. In many areas where it is not found naturally, it is added to the water supply to reduce dental decay. It can be taken as a supplement, but it can mottle or stain the teeth.

Foods containing fluoride (besides fluoridated water): canned salmon and sardines with bones.

Iron, ferrous sulfate. Iron is necessary for hemoglobin, the oxygen transporting protein in red blood cells. Unless directed by a doctor, it is recommended that men and postmenopausal women take multivitamins with little or no iron. Iron supplements cause constipation.

Heme iron, better absorbed than nonheme iron, comes from meat, poultry, ham, tuna. Nonheme iron comes from plant sources such as raisins, peas, lentils, figs, oatmeal, grits.

Magnesium. This mineral works with many enzymes to regulate body temperature, allow nerves and muscles to contract, and synthesize proteins.

Foods containing magnesium: fish, nuts, potatoes, legumes, whole grains, vegetables. Green vegetables are good sources because the center of the chlorophyll molecule, which gives green vegetables their color, contains magnesium. When flour is refined, the magnesium-rich

germ and bran are removed. "Hard" tap water contains more minerals, including magnesium.

Phosphorus. Important for bone and soft tissue growth, phosphorous is
so prevalent in food that deficiency is rare.

Selenium. This is a trace mineral essential to the immune system and thyroid gland. It works with vitamin E as an antioxidant. Although people with RA tend to have low selenium levels, there is contradictory
evidence about whether selenium supplements are helpful. Selenium deficiency is rare. Since there is not agreement on the therapeutic value of selenium for RA, it's best to make sure your
multivitamin contains selenium.

Foods containing selenium: fish, whole grains, beans, nuts, brewer's
yeast, shrimp, crab, poultry, garlic.

Zinc. Zinc is important for wound healing, cell reproduction, tissue
growth, and scores of enzymatic reactions. Zinc levels are low in
some people with RA. Studies of zinc supplements for RA have had
varying results. The best bet is to take a multivitamin that contains
zinc, and include foods containing zinc in your diet.

Foods containing zinc: egg yolk, whole grains, legumes, meats, fish,
poultry, soybeans, lentils, dairy products, pure maple syrup, peanut
butter, tofu, oysters, mussels, lobster.

Multiple vitamins

It's best to get your vitamins from food. But to hedge your bets, take a
multiple vitamin/mineral pill (MVM) as well. Beyond convenience, a multiple vitamin has a number of advantages. It gives you a range of vitamins
and minerals, filling in what you may not have gotten from diet alone. It is
more common to have an overall nutritional deficiency than a specific one.

In general, the comparisons on the label to the DV are useful when you
take into account that it is based on a 2,000-calorie diet. If you're female
and postmenopausal, you need more calcium and vitamin D to protect
against osteoporosis. Some minerals in higher doses, like calcium, would
increase the size of the tablet until it would be too big to swallow, so you
may want to take a separate supplement.

Although dosages vary with age and sex, specialized formulas for women,
seniors, and men are not regulated, so each company decides what goes into

a vitamin. Most formulas for women have added calcium, but check to see that they have the DV, based on a 2,000-calorie diet, against your caloric intake.

Store brands are likely to be as good as name brands, only much lower in price. Read the label, check the expiration date, and avoid added fillers and coloring agents.

Vitamins tend to work with other nutrients; take a supplement with meals. And raise a toast to your good health with a glass of carrot juice.

IN A SENTENCE:

> *A diet rich in vitamins and minerals can better replenish deficiencies, often found in RA, than supplements—although a daily vitamin is a wise safeguard.*

living

Considering Alternative Therapies

For better or for worse, nearly half of all Americans have used some kind of alternative therapy—also called complementary and alternative medicine (CAM). Some people are looking outside the medical profession out of frustration with a chronic condition, with the impersonality of managed care, or with the expense of treatment—particularly the uninsured.

The medical profession, contrary to its reputation for discrediting alternative practices, has brought many alternative practices that have been proven to be beneficial into the mainstream; it actively supports ongoing clinical trials and safety testing for others, as well as education about harmful therapies. Although no alternative therapy has been found to cure chronic conditions like RA, hospital pain clinics routinely use formerly alternative practices, including visualization and yoga. Relaxation techniques administered by psychologists are recognized by Medicare. If an alternative therapy is scientifically proven to be effective, it is no longer considered alternative.

However, some alternative therapies have been proven to have problematic interactions with other medications, other negative side effects, toxic contents, or unregulated dosages. Others remain untested, although the long process is under way.

Grasping at straws

Many of us, at some point in the progress of this disease, will try anything. Management of RA takes so much effort and patience that it is the rare person who will not reach out in hope for alternative cures. You might expect that scientifically unproven remedies would be used mainly by the less educated, but one study showed a majority of those drawn to them to be educated people. Normally discerning minds see relief in a testimonial the way a thirsty man sees a lake on the desert—a mirage created by desperation.

Bedridden with raging RA, I descended into the nether world of nostrums, tonics, and unctions, where anything is possible. Unseen throngs have been cured of rheumatoid arthritis with these elixirs—all sworn to by someone who knows someone else or who learned it on the Internet. Lazarus-like, they have all risen to do pliés and tangos and open car doors. They are skiing K-2 and cartwheeling and turning on their faucets. They are playing bocce ball and Ping-Pong and staying awake all day long. To hear it told, these people with their copper enzymes, alkaline balances, and chicken sternums are all out there doing whatever they want. And none of it worked for me. Much of it doesn't work for anyone else, either. The question is, which alternative therapies are safe and effective?

The Yellow Volkswagen Cure

I kept asking my rheumatologist about new potions. He said that because the disease waxes and wanes, a patient can be convinced that a remedy works when in fact the RA is naturally abating. "You may as well feel better when you see a yellow Volkswagen," he said. On the way home I saw two yellow Volkswagens, and I felt better right away. I've kept my eye out ever since, and found that the irony of pretending that it is a real cure makes me laugh, lifts my spirits, and works, well, like a talisman.

Bogus cures

Miracle cures flock to incurable diseases like metal filings to a magnet. Arthritis patients spend billions every year on untested remedies. More important than the waste of money for people with RA is the waste of time, because the earlier the intervention, the better chance we have of controlling the disease.

You can find enthusiastic accounts of RA cures—eating gin-soaked raisins, capsules of ground up ants, vinegar and honey, New Zealand green-lipped mussels; sitting in abandoned uranium mines, covering yourself in cow manure twice daily, standing naked under a full moon, keeping two sesame seeds in your navel overnight; wearing radioactive devices, copper bracelets, magnets; rubbing WD-40 on your joints (hey, it works for door hinges).

Other widely touted remedies deserving a healthy dose of skepticism, cited by The Harvard Medical School Arthritis Action Program, are: CMO, bromelain, DMSO (found in paint thinner), and MSM. These, as well as coenzyme Q10, are not scientifically proven to be of help, and some are known or suspected to be harmful.

Categories of alternative therapies

Alternative therapies are divided into five categories by the National Center for Complementary and Alternative Medicine (NCCAM, an agency within the NIH), followed here by a mix of proven and unproven examples.

Alternative medical systems: Chinese medicine, Ayurvedic medicine, homeopathy.
Mind-body practices: meditation, visualization, spiritual healing.
Biologic-based therapies: herbal medicines, dietary supplements, special diets.
Body-based therapies: massage, chiropractic, osteopathy.
Energy therapies: Reiki, therapeutic touch.

Sorting help from hype

Regulation, and therefore oversight, of alternative medical systems—such as Chinese and Ayurvedic medicine, as well as herbal remedies, vitamins, and nutritional supplements—has been hampered by a law permitting many remedies to be classified as dietary supplements. Although these products are pharmacologically active, they are exempt from the safety and efficacy requirements of prescription drugs, which are monitored by the Food and Drug Administration.

Several agencies, public and private, are studying the purity and efficacy of alternative remedies. Controlled trials are conducted by NCCAM. The government Integrated Neural Immune program is dedicated to studying mind-body practices. Over the last five years other research centers have increased testing.

So much variation has been found that this is a healthy area for skepticism. Watch for these signs of wishful thinking:

Secret formula. Legitimate scientists share knowledge in a peer review process, and results of research are published in journals.

Cure. Bona fide research toward a cure is known throughout the field. We will know if a potential cure is found long before it is available on the market. Read the fine print; there is apt to be a disclaimer.

Miraculous breakthrough. Testing is a long, slow process to approval, and again, such a finding would be subject to peer review. RA is complex and requires multiple treatment strategies.

Limited time only. Approved therapies are continually available. Any shortage of supplies, such as one during the start-up in manufacturing of a new biologic drug, is public information.

Recommended by doctors. Who are the doctors? Do they have a financial investment in the product? Is the product backed by professional societies like the American College of Rheumatology?

No mentioned side effects. All drugs have side effects; it is a matter of weighing the benefits against the disadvantages. Full information is listed on a bona fide package.

Treatment publicized by television infomercials, direct mail, telemarketing, newspaper ads pretending to be stories. Real treatment is first reported in medical journals.

Proof relying solely on testimonials. Regulated trials are done to prove the value and safety of medicines.

Clinically proven. Look for a mention of the publication of results of trials in a medical journal such as *The New England Journal of Medicine* or *Arthritis and Rheumatism*. Such a study would be over a long period with substantial numbers of subjects and a control group. The funding needs to come from sources without a vested interest in the outcome. More than one study should show the same result.

Ancient cure. Anesthesia used to be a knock on the head, and bloodletting was standard for fever; just because it was medical practice a long time ago does not make it better. Also, herbs touted for centuries can interact with modern medication.

Be wary of health practitioners who promise an outcome, do not have a diploma from a certified program, require you to pay a large amount in advance, tell you to quit your medications, claim your RA is caused by a food, or want you to keep the treatment secret. You must taper off some medications, such as cortisone.

Before you choose an alternative therapy, ask yourself if the source of information is reliable, what scientific basis is offered, and whether the cost is reimbursable through your insurance.

Checking in, keeping track, and staying aware

If you do decide to try an alternative treatment, it is important to check with your physician. It bears emphasizing that particular herbs can have harmful interactions with prescription medications, and patients must taper off some drugs. Don't let anticipation of hubris stop you from bringing up the subject. I have just spoken with a woman who was afraid to report to her doctor that she was trying a remedy that required her to be off medication. She knew her cortisone had to be tapered off and assumed that the next lowest number to one tablet was zero. Instead of lowering it by small fractions, as required for the adrenal glands to become active again, she stopped, and has suffered health consequences for years since.

There's a lot to remember; keep track of treatments and how you are feeling in your medical journal. You may be surprised to see patterns develop. For example, when I tried acupuncture, the practitioner would also do acupressure on the days when a client was not waiting. Looking at the chart, I saw that I felt soothed on the acupressure days and switched to massage that incorporated that technique.

Be careful that your information comes from reputable sources. I tried many cures that turned out to have no substance, and I can share this advice: Stay critical. Caveat emptor—buyer beware.

IN A SENTENCE:

> *Effective alternative therapies for RA have now become mainstream, while others are being tested, and many are dangerous in combination or are shams.*

learning

Specific Alternative Therapies

Many alternatives to choose from

So much of this is unmapped territory; venture into it with the guidance of your doctor. I have divided several categories of alternative therapies into those externally applied and those taken internally. The safest are those that are not ingested. This partial list includes those most often recommended for RA and some that are ill-advisedly used.

Noninvasive alternative treatments

MIND-BODY TECHNIQUES
Passive practices (like meditation, biofeedback, and visualization) and active practices (like yoga and tai chi) are the most commonly used and most effective alternative therapies for people with RA. (See Month 5.)

HEAT AND COLD

At one time rheumatology treatment was centered at spas because people believed in the healing power of warm water. There is no evidence that applied temperature change provides other than comfort and short-term relief. That is enough for most of us to use it regularly. Try a hot shower or bath, sauna, hot tub, warm towels, or heating pads.

Some people use peat baths or warm wax immersion. Wax baths for the hands, feet, or elbows were once used more than they are now; the joint is submerged in a melted wax and mineral oil until a thick coating is formed and then covered to retain heat. The bath itself has not been proven to do more than soothe, but there is some evidence that exercise of the warmed joints may be of help. My friend Nancy Etchemendy likes the treatment so much that she bought a home device to melt the wax.

Ice can give relief when applied to an inflamed joint for ten minutes or so several times a day. The old bag of frozen peas trick allows the cold source to wrap around the joint. Many people find it helpful to alternate heat and cold, but that appears to be a personal preference.

Caution: Don't place a heat source or ice directly on the skin or keep it in one place longer than twenty minutes. Don't use this therapy if you have cardiovascular problems.

MASSAGE

Massage has numerous benefits, not the least of which is the relaxing power of human touch. It increases circulation to tense muscles, improves joint movement, decreases stress hormones, and may help block pain signals.

You can massage your own joints with a few drops of oil. If you choose professional treatment, find a licensed masseuse, determine the cost, and learn whether it qualifies for insurance coverage. There are a number of practices—Swedish and Feldenkrais, for example. Discuss any treatment with your doctor, especially stronger massage techniques like Traeger, Shiatsu, Hellerwork, and Rolfing. I did try a gentler form of Rolfing, called Aston-Patterning, at a point when nothing was helping.

ACUPUNCTURE

It may take some suspension of disbelief to believe that a point near your elbow regulates immune function. Whatever the active mechanism, enough research has been done to show that acupuncture can help control arthritis pain. For some patients, relief is more immediate than for others. Study results for other RA symptoms are mixed. Acupuncturists are licensed in thirty-eight states. If you choose to try acupuncture, be certain that disposable needles are used.

Acupressure

Points on the body are stimulated by several minutes of pressure with the fingers. This treatment may also help to relax muscles and block pain signals

Ayurveda

Ayurveda is an Indian system of wellness-based practices, some of which can work with conventional medicine, such as yoga, meditation, and breathing exercises; eating a well-balanced vegetarian diet low in fats and rich in fruits and vegetables; setting up a daily routine that includes exercise, regular sleep, and reduced stress.

Be careful with herbs, addressed below, and internal cleansing therapies, some of which use equipment that enters your body. There is no U.S. licensing process for such therapies. The noninvasive Ayurvedic practices are a version of the beneficial advice you have heard from your doctor.

Homeopathy

Studies of the effects of homeopathy on RA have shown varying results. The theory is "like cures like," with people given miniscule amounts of materials that would cause illness in larger amounts. Licensed doctors can practice homeopathy in Arizona, Nevada, and California. The medications are diluted, creating few risks apart from the potential time delay in starting conventional medications. If you decide to try this approach, consult a doctor; don't try it alone, in spite of the fact that the Internet is abuzz with recipes to follow based on such indications as your moral code.

Topical creams

BenGay is an example of an aspirin-based cream that is absorbed into the system through the skin. Be aware that aspirin entering the body by any means can have the same side effects. Cayenne or red pepper creams mask joint pain, but they can offer some relief. Be sure to wash your hands carefully before touching your eyes; take it from one who knows.

ELECTRICAL STIMULATION

There is no evidence to support the use of electrical stimulation in the management of rheumatoid arthritis. Faradic baths, which use water along with electrical current, do not appear to help.

LOW-LEVEL LASER THERAPY

Low-level laser therapy uses a light source that causes photochemical reactions thought to relieve pain. It appears to provide short-term relief for RA. No improvement has been found for inflammation or range of motion, and no data exist for long-term effects.

ULTRASOUND

A few limited studies appear to show that ultrasound applied in water increased grip strength in people with RA when compared to a placebo treatment.

APITHERAPY

Beekeepers are said not to have arthritis because of beestings, and there is a long history of applying stings as a cure. I tried the sting cure, enlisting my husband to hold each bee to my back with a pair of tweezers; I developed symptoms of anaphylaxis. As he fumbled with the epinephrine syringe, he was imagining the local redneck police chief arriving to say, "You were doing *what* to your wife?"

Many lists of sham cures list apitherapy, but a study cited in the medical journal *Arthritis and Rheumatism* suggests that melittin, a major component of bee venom, has anti-inflammatory properties. Studies are under way to further isolate potentially helpful chemicals in bee venom. In the meantime, proceed cautiously with this therapy under the guidance of a medical professional.

Don't swallow every claim

Herbs have a reputation as natural, benign, ancient cures. Many people turn to herbal remedies when they are not restored to health by pharmaceuticals, and sometimes take both.

Proceed with caution: Herbs are pharmacologically active; in short, they are drugs, although they are not regulated as such. They can be contaminated, inaccurately formulated, or toxic in combination with other medication.

Grown in soil, they may contain anything contained in soil—bacteria, heavy metals, pesticides. When the California Department of Public Health tested herbal products, they found that 32 percent contained heavy metals.

Dr. Alice Domar of the Harvard Medical School calls the lack of control over the quality and quantity of herbs in different capsules "really frightening." I asked the dean of the UC School of Pharmacology about a combination of herbs suggested for me at a health food store. She came up with a study that concluded that the dosage recommended by the affable young clerk was toxic.

Herbal products are tested for safety and efficacy in controlled trials at the University of California Drug Information Analysis Service. The director, Candy Tsourounis, warns that just because something is natural does not mean that it is safe; a natural therapy can cause liver damage. A supplement or herb can counteract the effects of a prescription medication or become harmful in combination. For example, St. John's wort may reduce the effectiveness of immunosuppressant drugs, and ginseng, when combined with aspirin, can lead to bleeding.

Looking for the mark of purity

Evaluation of the purity of herbs and supplements can be found on the Internet at sites such as those for Consumer Lab (www.Consumer Lab.com), where you will find informative articles as well as product summaries. You can find free useful information, and studies are available by subscription.

"Key Ingredients Missing in Some Arthritis Supplements" heads a typical article on the site. Consumer Lab cautions that although supplements can be legally marked "complex," "formula," or "blend" without listing the weight of each component, the label is often misleading as to the actual contents.

United States Pharmacopeia (USP, www.usp.org), a nonprofit organization, sets standards for drugs and supplements manufactured in the U.S. The USP mark on a label tells you that the product has been tested and the following results found: ingredients stated on the label are present in the declared amount, nutrients are effectively released when the product dissolves, and the product is free of harmful contaminants.

Once you know that what you bought is genuinely in the bottle, then comes the tricky question: does it help?

Herbal remedies

I had intended to create a definitive list of herbal remedies grouped by effectiveness, but the task is impossible—not only for me but for the agencies studying them. The opinions of reputable scientific sources can vary on the same supplement from, at best, an okay to a resounding no. Since my own fruitless adventures into ingested alternatives, I've become skeptical on the subject. The best way for me to call it, I think, is to err on the side of caution and cite any question raised by a reliable source.

It is important to consider any herb in the context of your program; many, like echinacea, evening primrose oil, and bromelain, may interact with common prescription drugs. The effects of herbal supplements on a developing fetus are unknown, so if you are planning to become pregnant, it is not wise to take them. Following is a partial list of supplements commonly used for RA.

Bromelain

Bromelain is a substance derived from pineapples. It has not been tested for people with arthritis. The Harvard Medical School Arthritis Action Program states that there is not valid scientific evidence that it is an anti-inflammatory agent. Also, it may interact with common prescription drugs.

Chondroitin

Often found in combination with glucosomine, this popular supplement is usually derived from cow cartilage or that of pig, chicken, or shark. Some authorities conclude that there is no accepted scientific evidence that taking animal cartilage relieves any type of arthritis and no proof that this supplement reverses cartilage loss, as it is reputed to do. Others cite studies that suggest improvement in joint function. It has not been studied enough to know if it helps retain cartilage.

Medical anthropologists have described a pattern of consuming a like part of an animal to take on its attributes, like eating brain to become smart. It is the thinking of cannibals: eat someone powerful and become powerful. By that theory, I'd have done well to have taken a bite out of my rheumatologist's knee. Still, the possibility of helpful attributes is enough for the NIH to create a study of chondroitin in OA, which is now under way. Europeans have used the supplement for years.

Chondroitin is an expensive material, and Consumer Lab has found considerable variation in the quality and quantity marketed. One product, among many found wanting, contained 18 percent of the stated amount. Be careful with this supplement if you are taking blood thinners.

COPPER

Despite the popularity of copper cures for arthritis, it has not been proven that they work. Copper is a necessary mineral for general health, and it can be derived from food and vitamins. There are inconclusive studies in which people who wore copper bracelets said they got relief. It appears not to be a harmful practice.

DEVIL'S CLAW (HARPAGOPHYTUM PROCUMBENS)

This popular treatment for arthritis in Europe comes from an African plant. The roots contain a chemical that has anti-inflammatory and pain-killing properties shown in some studies to help OA symptoms. There is no evidence at this time that it helps RA.

DMSO

DMSO is a chemical solvent found in paint thinner, and is advertised as a topical anti-inflammatory. There have been few studies and conflicting results, and the supplement was found to cause a range of adverse reactions. The Harvard Medical School Arthritis Action Program finds that the commercial product is seldom pure.

FISH OIL

Some essential fatty acids, such as eicosapentaenoic acid found in fish oil, have been shown to ease arthritis symptoms in some people. They appear to provide building blocks for anti-inflammatory agents. If you take fish oil capsules, they can thin the blood and intensify the side effects of NSAIDs.

FLAXSEED

Flaxseed is high in an omega-3 fatty acid, which is known to be anti-inflammatory, but there are no conclusive studies to show that it eases arthritis symptoms. It is a natural laxative and can act as a blood thinner when taken in high amounts as a supplement. Flaxseed oil or flax seeds can be used in salads.

GIN-SOAKED RAISINS

This folk remedy may have come out of the fact that grapes and raisins do contain anti-inflammatory components. You can detour into detailed cybertheories that specify the number of raisins, but there is no clinical proof that it helps. Unless alcohol is contraindicated for a medication you take, you might be better off with a grape in a martini.

GINGER

Ginger is reported in some lab studies to relieve inflammation and pain. It is not known what effect it has on RA, but in one study it produced relief from joint pain in OA when taken with ibuprofen. Too much causes gastrointestinal problems or blood thinning. Use it in cooking or make it into tea.

GLA (GAMMA LINOLENIC ACID), EVENING PRIMROSE OIL, BORAGE OIL

Although there is evidence that GLA reduces inflammation in RA, some sources warn that it is better to get the oil nutritionally. Evening primrose oil may interact with common prescription drugs. (This is the remedy I was inquiring about when my rheumatologist suggested that I would be as well off feeling better when I saw a yellow VW.)

GLUCOSAMINE

This component of cartilage extracted from crab, lobster, and shrimp shells has been advertised as an arthritis cure. It is not a cure. It has been used in veterinary medicine for degenerative joint diseases in animals. A current study is being conducted by the NIH on people with OA, not RA. According to Dr. Kenneth Sack of the University of California at San Francisco, there is not sufficient evidence to show that it builds cartilage in either disease. Glucosamine is taken by supplement, as it is not found in food. Don't take it if you are allergic to shellfish.

GREEN TEA

Animal studies show it may be helpful to arthritis. It contains polyphenols, which are antioxidant compounds shown to reduce inflammation.

It seems to be safe, although some people are allergic to it. You could substitute it for coffee, as it has caffeine, or try decaffeinated green tea. If you want the equivalent given to the grateful mice whose arthritic symptoms subsided, try three to four cups a day.

MSM

MSM is used in veterinary medicine, but no studies have been done on people. It is derived from DMSO, which creates questions of purity. It is proposed for treating arthritis as well as snoring, dry skin, brittle nails, and cancer.

SAM OR SAME (S-ADENOSYLMETHIONINE)

SAM is produced naturally by eating green leafy vegetables. It helps with cartilage regeneration as well as neurotransmitters that affect mood. SAM supplements have long been used in Europe for, among other problems, OA. In one study it appears to alleviate moderate OA pain. No evidence of efficacy with RA is available. SAM supplements counteract methotrexate, may interact with antidepressants, and worsen Parkinson's disease. The best approach may be to eat dark leafy vegetables to promote natural SAM production.

STINGING NETTLE (URTICA DIOCA)

There is marginal evidence that stinging yourself with nettles on painful joints will reduce pain, and at least it will distract you. German studies suggest that eating nettles can possibly improve pain and stiffness, but talk to your doctor before you start to brew them up.

THUNDER GOD VINE (TRIPTERYGIUM WILFORDII)

This Chinese immunosuppressant was found, in a small NIH study, to improve the number of inflamed joints among people with RA. Further studies are needed to show whether or not it is safe and effective. Leaves and flowers are highly toxic; preparations under study come from the root only.

TURMERIC (CURCUMA LONGA, CURCUMA DOMESTICA)

Turmeric, an ingredient in curry powder, is traditionally used in Chinese and Ayurvedic medicine for arthritis. Few clinical studies have been done, but it has been shown to have anti-inflammatory properties. In high amounts it can thin the blood, but a dish of curry makes a pleasant dose.

WILLOW BARK

Willow bark has the same active ingredient as aspirin: salicylic acid. You'd need a lot of cups of willow bark tea to get the equivalent of one aspirin tablet, and supplement products vary with the species and preparation. The benefits and adverse side effects are the same as they are for aspirin.

VITAMINS

People with arthritis often have vitamin and mineral deficiencies, thought to be a result of the disease or medication rather than the cause. It's best to get an adequate intake of vitamins and minerals through your diet and a standard daily vitamin. (See Month 3.)

IN A SENTENCE:

Noninvasive alternative practices can be safer choices for RA management than other remedies, which need to be reviewed with a doctor for potential impurity, toxicity, or interference with prescription medication.

living

Sleep, Rest, and Relaxation

> *Sometimes, Lord, you got to relax your mind.*
> —LEADBELLY

Relaxation influences immune function

The line blurs in RA between physical stress on the joints and emotional stress from having a chronic condition; one triggers the other in a cycle of increasing joint pain. With active RA, it is important to set aside time during the day to alleviate both kinds of stress.

You can lessen the physical stress of the disease with enough rest and sleep. The emotional stress dissolves with mind-body practices that create physiologic change, such as meditation.

Researchers are examining the relationship between the levels of damaging cortisol production in RA and control of external daily stressors. "The processes that fire up the immune system and lead to the proliferation of inflammation-inducing chemicals are the same processes that are stimulated by stress," according to Dr. Alex Zautra, an arthritis researcher at Arizona State University. Stress reduction techniques, many of which are discussed in Day 2, have been shown to help restore the balance in your system.

As my mother-in-law reminds me, it's not what you go through, it's how you go through it. It sounds too good to be true—no-cost, drug-free, non-invasive ways to deal with RA. Not all of these disciplines are equally suited to everyone, but they are doors into the same room.

You snooze, you win

Make rest part of your daily schedule in order to manage the fatigue that comes with RA. Plan to lie down twice a day for fifteen to thirty minutes, or as you need it. You will recover better if you rest regularly before you become depleted. When RA fatigue is ignored, it can take a long time, days even, to come back from exhaustion. Most people find that the need for daily rest declines as they take care of themselves.

If you are in a demanding job with little opportunity to rest, it would be wise to reconsider your schedule or even your job. It may take some inventiveness or the jettisoning of some pride to arrange a place to nap.

Midafternoon is a time when energy often wanes, but individual patterns vary. A review of your journal notes can be revealing; fatigue can be associated with particular kinds of stressful work, too. Balance physical activity, say a walk at lunchtime, with an afternoon rest period and perhaps rest after work.

Sleep

There are compelling reasons for those of us with RA to plan for proper rest at night. Lack of sleep wreaks havoc on the immune system. A recent study at Pennsylvania State University's Hershey Medical Center showed that the reduction of sleep in healthy college students to six hours for a week resulted in increases in cytokines, the inflammation-promoting chemical found in people with RA.

In sleep, metabolism slows and your body takes on the task of repairing bones and tissues. **REM (Rapid Eye Movement) sleep** is described as an alert mind in a paralyzed body, characterized by dreaming. In non-REM sleep, there is very low mental activity. Lack of REM sleep is associated with night awakenings and restlessness as well as with food cravings. Sleep deprivation can interfere with the modulation of pain. Information is processed during sleep; you can go to bed with a problem and awake with new ideas.

"Sleep macho" is what one therapist calls the respect in our culture for people who function on little sleep. Over the last century, we've cut our average sleep time by about 30 percent. On the other hand, it is not clear that more sleep means better health; there can be too much sleep. The balance is individual, with seven to eight hours often cited as optimal and some people normally sleeping as much as ten, like Albert Einstein. To know how much you need, observe yourself on vacation—when you become drowsy and when you awaken on your own. Many people need more sleep when RA is active.

In a nationwide sleep poll, 72 percent of people with arthritis reported sleep problems. Fatigue is a frequent symptom of sleep disturbances, but it is not to be confused with sleepiness. Women are about 10 percent more likely than men to have insomnia. Stress can interrupt sleep, and lack of sleep causes stress, leading to insomnia—a downward cycle. With lack of sleep your reaction time slows, and you become absentminded. After being awake for seventeen hours, you perform at the level of a blood alcohol of .05, almost legally drunk. Regular sleep is necessary for managing RA. If you are having trouble sleeping, consider these suggestions:

Exercise produces deep, restorative sleep, but don't schedule exercise near bedtime.

Maintain a regular sleep schedule. I call this my George Washington policy. Historians say he would rise at a dinner party in his own house, and invite people to carry on without him as he excused himself, saying it was his bedtime. Going to bed and getting up at the same time every day is a form of conditioning, according to Dr. Clete Kushida, director of the Stanford University Center for Human Sleep Research. He suggests sleeping in on weekends no more than an extra hour to maintain the pattern.

If you can't sleep, get up. Dr. Kushida suggests that after twenty minutes of tossing, get up and do something relaxing for a while—drink herbal tea or read.

Use relaxation techniques. Try progressive relaxation, described below. A study at Harvard Medical School showed that meditation and breathing techniques, in this case those in kundalini yoga, improved sleep.

Avoid caffeine (coffee, tea, soft drinks, chocolate) for several hours before bed. This varies with the individual, but caffeine can be in your system for twelve hours. For most people, the maximum is two cups of coffee before noon.

Moderate alcohol for several hours before bed. The nightcap is misnamed; it may make you feel sleepy at first, but it will suppress REM sleep, making your sleep less deep and more erratic. You will wake up more tired as a result.

Take a warm bath or shower. The warmth is relaxing.

Turn off technology; it encourages you to stay up late and wakes you up early. Pick a time to stop taking incoming calls and shut off the television. Plan a quiet activity before bed.

Put the pets out. The Mayo Clinic reports that pets in the bedroom disrupt the sleep of 53 percent of their owners.

Create a bedtime routine. It puts your mind at rest that you are prepared for the next day and gives a Pavlovian signal that it is time to wind down for sleep. Put a pad of paper next to your bed to jot down things that you are tempted to get up and do.

Keep your room cool. A lower temperature, about 67 degrees Fahrenheit, will lower your body temperature and slow your metabolism, helping you to sleep.

Darken your room. Try window shades or a sleep mask. Light can lower your body's melatonin level and keep you awake.

In addition, the quality of your sleeping space can influence your rest. Choose a firm or semifirm mattress. Some people with RA prefer memory foam or adjustable air mattresses. Make yourself at home in the mattress store, trying different sleeping positions before you make a selection. If you have trouble rising from a chair, consider increasing the height of the bed to the bottom of your buttocks when you stand. You can adjust the surface height with additional layers, such as memory foam. Turning and rotating the mattress will extend its life.

Pull your pillow all the way to your shoulder to support your neck. Consider an orthopedic pillow. A body pillow placed between inflamed knees can be helpful. It became a joke when a friend and I were bedridden with RA, but it's true that satin sheets make turning over easier when you are really hurting.

Mindfulness

Mindfulness is a term you will hear in connection with mind-body practices. It is not mystical; it simply means paying attention, being present and aware— observing without judgment. It is the opposite of the "monkey-mind," which is what Buddhists call the internal chatter that makes it difficult to focus— jumping between reruns from the past to anxiety for the future. The goal of these practices is not to reach nirvana but to quiet the mind noise so that you can watch from the stands. You will see that stress does not have you in its grip; you have stress in your grip. You can learn a process to let it go.

This inner awareness has been shown to be useful with chronic illness. Such practices have a biological impact on the brain. The Maryland Center for Integrative Medicine is currently tracking the relationship of these practices to inflammation, including gene expression, in patients with RA.

Thinking your way out

In Day 2 there is discussion of many ways to deal with psychological stress, including patterns of thinking. Negative thought can be dissolved with mind-body practices as well. Mindfulness-Based Stress Reduction (MBSR) is a program designed to teach people to recognize stressful thoughts and let them drift away. The program is directed by Trish Magyari, at the Center for Integrative Medicine at the University of Maryland Medical Center, who says, "People learn that self-defeating thoughts are doorways to the pit of their own personal despair. If they can learn to see the doorway, they can learn they don't have to go through it."

The relaxation response

The relaxation response is a measurable state of calm in which your blood pressure drops, your heart and breathing rate slow, and your muscles release tension. The technique was developed by Dr. Herbert Benson at Harvard in the early 1970s, and he has written a number of books on the subject. He is now the head of the Mind/Body Institute. Learning to trigger the relaxation response in your body is not an esoteric discipline; you can learn it the way you learn to type—by practice (which is why these are called "practices"). There are simple ways to acquire this skill, through meditation, deep breathing, visualization, or biofeedback—to name a few.

Whatever practice you choose, you will need a quiet environment, one in which you won't be disturbed. You will need to come to it with a passive attitude; it's not a job to be done or a goal to be accomplished. It is the opposite of doing; it is undoing. Don't strive to do it successfully; doing it is success, whatever the experience.

Stress relievers

I know people for whom a lot of these ideas are just too weird. Mindfulness is not patented by the Buddhists. You can string green beans mindfully. You can be in a meditative state with any activity that gets you into a frame of mind called flow, a feeling of being completely engrossed—familiar to athletes as being "in the zone," but just as much a part of the lives of musicians, quilters, or anyone who loses himself in a favorite pursuit. It appears that repetitive activity can trigger the relaxation response—bicycling, walking, jogging, playing a musical instrument, knitting, doing tai chi, or uttering repeated prayer. It's not so far out; it's far in.

Integrative clinics

The federal government's Integrated Neural Immune Program is dedicated to mind-body research.

Clinics that treat pain and stress with alternative techniques can be found at some teaching hospitals. There are over thirty in the U.S, including the Duke Center for Integrative Medicine in Durham, North Carolina, and the University of California Osher Center for Integrative Medicine in San Francisco. At the Center for Mindfulness in Medicine, Health Care and Society at the University of Massachusetts Medical School, 15,000 people have taken an eight-week course in meditation. These clinics use a variety of practices, including biofeedback, acupuncture, visualization exercises, mediation, and yoga. Check with your insurance to see what treatments are covered.

IN A SENTENCE:

> *Adequate rest, sleep, and relaxation play a key role in the physiology of RA.*

learning

Meditation Practices

The quieter you become, the more you can hear.
— RAM DASS

Breathing techniques

Breathing takes care of itself, but paying attention to the way we breathe can serve us well. Pain and stress interfere with breathing patterns, with respiration quickening even in the anticipation of discomfort. Deep abdominal breathing is used in many relaxation techniques; it can alter your psychological state.

Try it. Place one hand on your abdomen below your breastbone. Close your eyes and become aware of your breath, slowly inhaling through your nose and exhaling through your lips. Breathe deeply, filling your diaphragm. Take care not to breathe so quickly and deeply that you hyperventilate, becoming lightheaded from too much oxygen and not enough carbon dioxide.

You can make it a practice for ten or fifteen minutes every morning or evening. It's a good trick to use for stressful moments. A few slow, deep breaths before you speak can prevent a good measure of regret.

Progressive relaxation

The theory behind the technique called progressive relaxation, or Jacobson's progressive relaxation, is that accentuating physical tension helps in effecting its release. It is simply accomplished; tense a muscle group and then let go. It works.

Set aside fifteen to twenty minutes for this exercise. You can do this lying down, at your desk, on a plane. Keep your body in place and sequentially alter the tension in your muscles. Start with your feet, slowly pulling them up as though you are going to lift your toes, and release. In the same way tighten your calves, then your thighs and buttocks, and then your abdominal and chest muscles, releasing each in turn. Stretch your fingers straight, relax, and continue with your arm muscles. Press your shoulder blades together, tightening the upper back and neck before letting go. Do the same with your jaw and forehead. As you move through the practice, breathe deeply and evenly, allowing each muscle group to go limp.

Another way of using this technique is the body scan; quietly take inventory of your body, selectively stopping where you feel tension, increasing the tension and releasing it. The practice helps decrease stress and improves sleep. It is good to do in bed at the end of the day. I have found that it makes me much more aware of areas of my body that are tense, and I am always surprised to discover my jaw clenched, my brow furrowed, or my neck tight. This practice has not stopped my muscle tension; like debris on a riverbank, it always seems to gather at the same places. I have learned, though, to recognize and release it.

Meditation

Meditation has been well studied. The purpose is to quiet the mind, and in so doing, meditation quiets the body as well. Its measurable alpha brain wave patterns affect physical processes. Brain scans suggest that the training of the mind reshapes the brain to reduce stress. A number of studies show that meditation can ease arthritic symptoms.

Once consigned to the counterculture, meditation has become an accepted therapy. Some form is practiced by ten million Americans. It is a key element in the Arthritis Self-Help Course at Stanford University, which has been taken by over 100,000 people.

Meditation has brought me through times of pain, anguish, loss, and hopelessness. Some days it winnows out needless frustrations from the things that matter, leaving me feeling like I've shed a burden when I get up.

The writer Alice Walker, who has been meditating for some twenty years, describes her experience: "I felt myself drop into a completely different internal space. A space filled with the purest quiet, the most radiant peacefulness . . . what I'd got was that meditation took me right back to my favorite place in childhood: gazing out into the landscape, merging with it and disappearing."

Meditation is not a religious practice, although it has been part of almost every world religion since antiquity. It is a portable tool, at home with your own religious or spiritual beliefs. It is the work of a lifetime and of the moment. Don't save it for the hard times—it's a process that is part of your life. The calm lucidity of mind that comes with meditation creates perspective, compared with a stressful internal chaos that reacts to life.

Anyone can do it. Sit quietly in a comfortable position. Traditionally, you sit on the floor cross-legged with your buttocks raised by a firm cushion, which helps straighten your back. Just assume a position that feels best, and don't be daunted by proper form. Sit in a chair or even lie down if you need to. Relax.

Breathe deeply and sit with your shoulders softly back and your spine straight—a stance of relaxed attention. Bring your focus to your breathing. When your mind wanders, allow the thought to pass through without engaging, and come back to your breathing. At first it may seem impossible for more than a moment. Just observe that without judgment. Stick with it, even when it doesn't seem to be working; the practice of watching your mind is the way it works. Sometimes it can be agonizing to sit with your mind racing, and even harder to accept that it's fine, that observing it is all you are doing. Don't try to change anything. It is the process that is important. Just watch yourself running after and away from thoughts and let them go. The Buddhists call this "monkey mind"; one teacher calls it "puppy mind"—sniffing everything that comes along. The attitude is one of acceptance, but it is not to be confused with resignation. We are used to thinking of a goal as something to strive for, not something that we allow to happen. When you pay attention in this way, the facts of your life don't change, but the stress of struggle subsides. When you finish, sit quietly for a moment before you get up.

If your joints are too uncomfortable for you sit for long, you can try walking meditation. Pace slowly in a quiet place, focusing on your breath. If you wish, you can divide the time between sitting and walking until you find a comfortable combination. The process is the same—suspending judgment, focusing on your breath, and allowing the traffic of the mind to go by without joining it

Some people meditate with a mantra, an ancient practice of repeating a word or phrase that occupies the mind. You can choose a short phrase or prayer that is rooted in your belief. Breathe slowly and say the words as you exhale. Many find it helps with focus. I learned by counting breaths, with each inhalation a number up to ten. The idea is, when the mind wanders, to put the puppy back on the newspaper. It's important to be patient with your practice. After all, you are changing ingrained habits of your mind.

Meditation is most beneficial if it is done daily. You will find that the benefits creep into your life invisibly. Even five or ten minutes of deep relaxation can leave you calm and renewed. Increase to twenty minutes as you can. Once you have a meditation practice, you can meditate unobtrusively anywhere—waiting in the airport or in the doctor's office.

With this much, you can start your practice. You can learn more about meditation from books and tapes. Jon Kabat-Zinn has written and recorded several. A group is helpful; there is quite a different feeling meditating with a group.

If you are considering a meditation retreat, research it carefully. Community centers, adult education programs, and hospitals often have non-religious meditation instruction. You may need to try more than one program to find one you like. If it is part of a stress-reduction program, it may be paid for by your insurance. Cost varies from free or a donation to the full professional fee of a therapist.

VISUALIZATION PRACTICES

If deep breathing is not the most ancient of these techniques, then visualization surely is. Prehistoric cave paintings are thought to picture successful hunts as preparation for the hunt. Modern sports trainers use visualization practices; Olympic athletes can be seen on camera before an event, eyes closed, arms going through the motions of, say, the pole vault. Seeing a desired result in the mind's eye helps create the outcome.

Visualization or guided imagery is used in psychotherapy, biofeedback, and stress-reduction programs. It is a safe, drug-free approach to relaxation and well worth a try. Most studies have examined visualization together with other relaxation techniques. They suggest, but do not prove, that the combination improves immune function.

You can learn a visualization practice in group or private sessions, or you can learn from a book or recording. Most sessions begin with deep breathing or other relaxation exercises. Your choice of visualization depends on your goal.

Find a quiet, comfortable place to sit. You can lie down if you like, but don't use the exercise as a way to induce sleep; the idea is to learn to relax while you are awake. If you can, schedule this the same time every day. If you start out with a recording, you can eventually create your own mind pictures and guide yourself through them.

These exercises work best when you allow your imagination to engage. If you visualize yourself on a beach, feel the sand on your feet, soft and hot, or wet, firm, and cold. Engage every sense. Smell the salt air, feel the breeze or stillness of the air. Look around, stretching your neck to see the sky, the clouds—particular clouds, gathering or dissipating. Sense your body as you move.

A number of visualization exercises that deal with pain picture it as melting, being pushed or drawn out of the body, or happening far away.

You can use visualization to rid yourself of the weight of anger, particularly if you are not ready to deal with a problem directly. Sit quietly and imagine yourself in a comfortable room, one with familiar and loved objects that you take time to examine. Bring someone you feel resentment toward to your door. Open it and invite the person in, noticing the emotions you feel that block his entrance. Choose a place for the person to sit and tell him silently that you forgive him. Breathe deeply, allowing yourself to let go of the resentment, and guide the person out the door.

In my experience, it can take a few times around for this to take effect. The stress of resentment, of course, belongs to the person who carries it. Obviously it would only intensify the problem to focus on a negative outcome. This exercise also works in asking forgiveness for yourself. Take note of the emotions that the process evokes.

The following exercise was taught to me years ago:

Imagine yourself outside, walking on a path in a familiar place that you love. Take your time and observe your surroundings—the sounds, warmth, colors, movement of the air, season of the year, very small living things. In the distance you can see something moving. As you walk, you see that it is a person approaching on the path, and it is some time before you recognize the person as yourself—yourself as you want to become. When you come face to face, you ask this self a question, an important question. You get a clear answer. You then ask this self to agree to become you for a moment, and when it does, it merges with your body. Now you are as you want to become. Sense how it feels—perhaps light, pain free, alert, joyful. Then separate your selves and ask if the other would consent to staying with you for the day as a consultant. With an affirmative answer, you can slowly come back and open your eyes.

There are many such tricks for telling yourself what you already know, and as you conduct your own guided imagery, you will become creative in finding some of your own.

Biofeedback

I had the opportunity see the power of biofeedback in a game at NextFest, a display of ingenious inventions in San Francisco. At either end of a long table, two players sat with electrodes on their heads. In the center of a groove that ran the length of the table rested a metal ball. The competitors quieted their minds, with their brain waves showing on a screen. The deeper the calm, the more alpha waves measured in the brain, the more the ball moved in the direction of a player until it reached one side or the other for a win. I tried it. Sure enough, as I allowed the relaxation response to take effect, the ball moved my way.

Early biofeedback experiments were done on Zen Buddhist monks in the 1950s with the intriguing finding that the hierarchy of brain waves matched the temple hierarchy of lay practitioners, monks, and teacher. Since that time, a number of body functions once thought to be involuntary have been shown to be possible to control. Biofeedback has become a tool used in pain clinics and therapy to teach techniques to improve pain, stress, anxiety, and sleep patterns.

Biofeedback involves being painlessly hooked up with sensors to a machine that monitors brain waves. You are taught to recognize thoughts that affect your body and are taught mental techniques—such as breathing, visualization, and meditation—to achieve physical results. The goal is for you to gain enough control to continue the practice on your own, without the equipment. The number of sessions it takes to accomplish this varies, as does the cost.

Contact the Biofeedback Certification Institute of America (www.bcia.org) to locate certified practitioners in your area. Some insurance may cover the cost, with a doctor's prescription.

Hypnosis

Hypnosis is very much like guided imagery. It is another technique to help focus attention and foster relaxation. Not all people are susceptible to hypnosis, perhaps as few as 25 percent. Hypnosis is described as a state in which one is aware of surroundings but deeply relaxed. Literature on hypnosis says that a hypnotized person will not accept unreasonable suggestions.

Autogenic training is a form of self-hypnosis that uses calming verbal suggestions or imagery.

Spiritual life

A spiritual life can both buoy and relax your mind, whether it is through a formal religion or not. Studies show that a spiritual outlook is helpful in adjusting to chronic disease. Many practices incorporate visualization, music, meditation, and prayer. Prayer, it has been found, can evoke the relaxation response.

Opening myself to the unexpected brought me rich experiences: An elderly Hispanic neighbor came to my bed and performed a healing rite—placing a picture of the stigmata on me. (It entered my mind that the picture best illustrated what this disease felt like at the time.) She prayed in mellifluous Spanish with such fervent faith that I was swept into the ecstasy of it. I envied such belief.

Another friend took me to walk the labyrinth in Grace Cathedral in San Francisco. A circular path, copied from Chartres Cathedral in France, winds back and forth in a pattern. In quiet, prayerful meditation, worshipers pace slowly into the center and back out. The ritual left me with an inexplicable sense of calm and joy.

You will find your own path, your own spiritual practice, your own way on a map that is as individual as your fingerprint and as universal as your hand.

IN A SENTENCE:

> *Calming the mind through various practices, such as meditation, has physiologic effects that benefit RA.*

living

Joint Protection and Adaptations

The protection racket—keeping joints safe

You may not have to give up things that you enjoy doing because of joint pain from RA if you learn to do them differently. Attention to body mechanics allows you to reduce the pressure on your joints to alleviate pain and reduce potential damage. Rest inflamed joints by taking breaks, varying your work, and using splints. Reduce the effort it takes to do a job by organizing your environment and using helpful devices.

Again, posture is key (see Week 4). Distribute your weight evenly by standing up straight. Put your shoulders softly back and pull up your spine, centering yourself over your feet, which should be about shoulder width apart. If you lean in different directions, you will find a sweet spot in the middle where you feel balanced and rooted. It is from that place that you will redistribute the stress on your joints when you engage with the world.

Distributing the pressure

Listening to your joints is a skill you pick up when you scan your body for tension. (See Month 5.) Respect the signals your body sends. You will begin to recognize when a joint starts to fatigue, allowing you to rest it before it becomes worse. You will also be able to distribute pressure on your joints in ways that avoid stressing them.

The rule of thumb, or of whole hand in this case, is to use the largest joint to do a job. Pick up a cup with both hands instead of an index finger, carry a plate with your hands, a tray on your forearms, a grocery bag encircled in your arms. Have some fun with it—closing a drawer with your foot, nudging a cupboard door with your shoulder, giving a door a bump with your butt. It adds up, or minuses down, reducing the stress on your joints.

You get the drift: Use the side of your hand on a spray can rather than a finger, carry a purse on your shoulder or use a backpack purse, use a flat hand to squeeze a sponge or wash a car, close containers with an elbow, insert your hand into a flat scrubber rather than gripping a brush, use both arms to hang clothes up, carry your briefcase on a padded shoulder strap. Wide-handled implements will help you shift pressure to larger joints.

Substitute lightweight objects where you can reduce joint stress—stainless steel for a cast-iron pan, for example, or dividing heavy bags, like flour or sugar, into smaller containers. Find ways other than lifting to move things—sliding, using wheels (a dolly is a useful tool).

When you must lift, instead of using your arms, use your whole body. Instead of your back, use your legs. Bend your legs, holding the object close to your body, lift smoothly with the legs. Don't lift heavy objects above your waist.

To pick up a child, lower yourself onto one knee, tighten your stomach muscles and hold the child close. Use your legs to lift.

Use the laws of physics to work for you, taking advantage of leverage when you can, like opening a flip-top can with a table knife.

To stand up from a chair, scoot forward, placing one foot forward and the other foot back. Rock forward, pushing up from the chair with your hands flat, palms down. A higher chair can help. A low easy chair can be frustratingly misnamed.

Choose to sit while working. A high stool is useful for the kitchen counter or workbench. Some people find it helpful to put one or both knees higher than the hips by placing their feet on a stool. If you need to stand to work, raise one foot on a low stool and alternate.

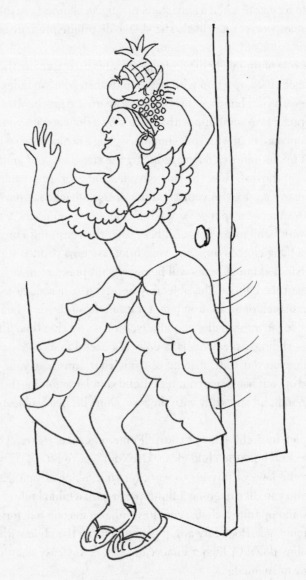

Use larger joints in daily routines, such as the cha cha door close.

The curse of the chopsticks

Even without RA, repeated use of small joints can cause damage. An example is shown in a study of 2,500 Beijing residents age sixty or older who use chopsticks. The results, sponsored by the National Institute of Arthritis and Musculoskeletal and Skin Diseases (NIAMS), showed that the repeated pinching pressure caused significant wearing of cartilage, which cushions the ends of bones, leading to joint pain and stiffness. Women tend to develop more hand OA than men, as was the case here. The point is not to eschew chopsticks, but to be aware of the need to shift stress to larger joints when possible to avoid adding to the mischief of RA.

Changing up; alternating activities

You will get more use out of your affected joints if you balance rest and work. Avoid staying in one position for an extended time. Avoid scheduling situations where you can't stop when you experience joint fatigue. Plan your rest periods into the day.

Divide work into smaller increments, and plan big jobs for the time of day when you are the most comfortable. Alternate tasks between sitting and standing, heavy and light.

When you sit, every once in a while stretch out each leg, flex your toes, write a few letters in the air. Flex your hands, too; squeeze a pliable ball, made for the purpose, while you are on the phone. When you take a break, scan your body for areas of gathered stress. Go through range-of-motion exercises to reduce the stress. You may find a period of meditation or visualization useful as well.

Simple choices to take strain off joints

Take the easy way to reduce the effort it takes for you to do a job: Use an electric toothbrush, microwave, electric can opener, food processor, blender, electric drill or screw driver. Tape record rather than take notes. Buy permanent press clothing.

Keep things where you use them, eliminating trips to get what you need. When you use something in more than one location, use duplicates.

Consider how hard the floors are where you stand to work. My downstairs laundry room is on a concrete floor and requires a thick rubber work mat.

Wearing gloves in the garden makes it easier to grip tools.

Make a joint warmer with a knotted sock full of rice or beans heated in the microwave. A sock can be cut to make an elbow warmer. Use a sleeping bag for your legs when reading or watching television.

Use a sharp knife at your place setting for meals, since it requires less pressure than a regular dinner knife. And save your precious index finger from pressing down on the knife by bringing your whole hand around the handle.

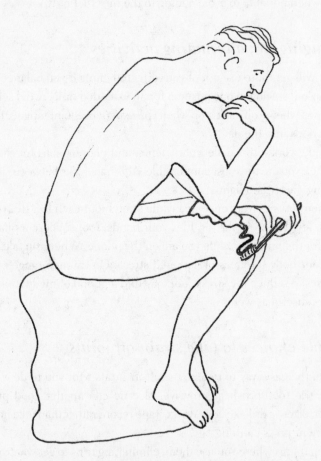

Use larger joints for small tasks when possible.

Getting your team to help

In a word: delegate. Those around you may be happier to lug groceries or roll up the rug than you suppose. It's good to spread the requests out rather than save up for an afternoon's labor. If you have a cooking companion, it makes food preparation easier and more enjoyable.

Teaching young children to pick up after themselves is a gift to you and to them as well. Keeping a limited number of toys accessible makes the job easier and refreshes interest in those toys that are rotated back for play. I need to remind my athletic sons and husband not to close lids too tightly.

Shaking hands

In business, many people feel that a firm handshake conveys confidence. In some churches, the pastor asks people to shake hands in welcome with those around them. A firm squeeze of the knuckles can be torture for tender joints, so it's wise to have a strategy before a smiling person approaches with outstretched hand.

My friend, the children's writer-illustrator Sarah Wilson, offers this advice: "My own choice is to slide past a person's open hand, ignore their palm, and encircle their wrist in a diplomatic arm clasp. This sometimes confuses people, but it works and even looks like it might be some kind of scouting tradition.

"When time allows, you also can touch or reach directly for the side of a person's hand, wrist or arm before a handshake. If someone insists on a traditional old-boy handshake, push into their palm and swivel your hand to encircle their thumb like the horn of a saddle, then release. This looks extremely strange and may cause startled expressions, but can work for hands which are only mildly painful." Best, she says, is to "wear something with pockets and keep your hands inside them. Nod and bow when necessary. Smile broadly."

I find that explaining the situation usually leads into the topic of RA (the uncle who had it in his thumb or the stinging nettle cure) if that is where you want to go. Mostly I try to duck between the hand buzzer and the filibuster with one of the halfway approaches or do an end-play and go for the cheek kiss.

Working at a desk

Choose a chair with a firm, straight back at a height that positions the work surface two inches below your elbows. If your work lends itself to using a drafting table as a tilted desk, you may prefer it. Sit tall without leaning forward.

When using a computer, avoid working with your laptop on your lap, which strains your neck. With the computer on a table, adjust the height of your chair until your arms are at 90 degrees to the keyboard and your eyes are level with the top third of the monitor. That will require you to elevate a laptop and use a separate keypad. It saves strain to use a document holder the same distance from your eyes as the screen. Headphones with a foot pedal for transcribing are useful, as is voice-activated software—said to have improved since I found it to produce more stress than sense. Keep your wrists soft; you may want to use a wrist rest. If your feet do not touch the floor, use a book, but not this one.

Once again, stretch often and stay aware of mounting muscle tension.

Driving

Sit close enough to the wheel so that your legs are flexed and comfortable. Add cushioning to your seat to help your posture. You may find a swivel seat helpful for getting in and out of the car. Key handles can help you turn on the ignition; I used to put a pen in the key ring to turn it. You can put a looped band around the door handle if you find closing it to be difficult.

Consider the effect on your joints of driving long distances and plan for rests.

If you are shopping for a car, check for the ease of using the control panel, various handles, side mirrors. The height of the seat will influence how easy it is to get in and out of the car.

Easy food preparation

If you are the family cook, fatigue at the end of the day can make shopping a chore and the kitchen seem like a dungeon. Eating right seems like a daunting undertaking when it is so easy to snack on unhealthy food. When your fingers ache, the last thing you want to do is chop vegetables.

Planning your menu for the week can take the pressure off your spirit and your joints. You'll generate a list that will make it easier to shop, and it will take one more thing off your mind. Choose meals that require a minimum of preparation. Convenience foods have become available with low salt, low fat, and few additives, but beware: read labels to see whether health-touting products are really calorie-laden junk foods. A wide variety of peeled and sliced fruits and vegetables can be found in most supermarkets, both fresh and frozen, to reduce stress on your hands. Canned foods are less appealing and nutritious, but they will do in a pinch.

When you do have time to cook, make double or triple amounts and freeze labeled portions. During the winter I make a Crock Pot of soup once a week; it smells good to come home to, is ready by dinner time, and provides leftovers, stored frozen in paper cups for lunch.

Take into account the effort to clean up when you plan meals. Line roasting pans with aluminum foil to make cleanup easier; it can be recycled. Occupational therapists are full of suggestions for making your life easier.

Some grocery stores deliver for a reasonable rate. You can also shop online for food and prescription medications. In many areas, weekly boxes of fresh organic vegetables are delivered from nearby farms.

Home environment

Rearrange your surroundings to make life easier; for example, position things for ready access, add roll-out shelves, and install a raised toilet seat. Levers are easier to use than doorknobs, which require grasping and turning. Lower closet racks reduce lifting. A control unit from a store like Radio Shack allows you to turn appliances on or off from one place. (See the following chapter for more aids.)

If you have the opportunity to structurally modify your home, or if you are moving and have a choice of locations, look for elements that will make it comfortable. Avoid hills, multiple staircases, and hard-to-reach cabinets. Carpeting or foam-backed rugs can help ease the strain on legs. Wheels on furniture make cleaning easier. Grab bars in the bathtub will help in lifting yourself. Abundant natural light will elevate your mood.

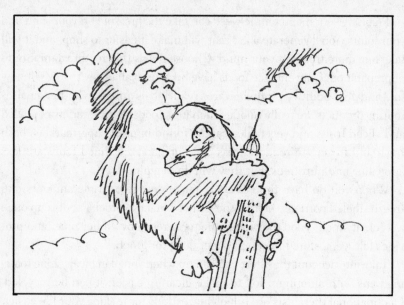

RIGHT: Distribute weight to large joints.

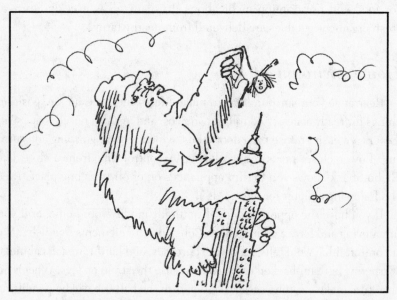

WRONG: Do not supend weight from small joints.

Insurance support for aids

Most insurance plans, including Medicare and Medicaid, are prepared to cover products and services that rehabilitate, when accompanied by a Certificate of Medical Necessity signed by a physician.

Oh, rats, there are limits

Repeated reaching and grasping tasks that mimicked human job-related movements in lab tests of rodents have shown an inflammatory response. The results resembled that of humans with musculoskeletal disorders from awkward positioning or stress injury. It may feel okay to suspend your purse from your forefinger while you juggle an armload of purchases to open the door, but invisible damage can be avoided in the small moments when you pause to do it right.

IN A SENTENCE:

> *You can minimize damage caused by physical stress on your joints by distributing weight through proper posture, shifting stress to larger joints, and using various aids.*

learning

Accommodating Your Needs

One hundred ways to work the world

All of your joints need protection, not just the tender, sore ones, because the effects of RA are systemic. Good posture and shifting stress to larger joints are important, but they may not be enough. Aids designed to absorb or adjust joint stress are particularly valuable for your smaller, more vulnerable joints. Numerous lightweight tools and utensils with a more open hand grip can be bought or made.

Twelve years ago, when I was diagnosed, a limited number of these aids were available, and only through specialty shops. Now that the boomers are starting to wear out, there is a far greater range of design and distribution. People who don't have arthritis are attracted to ergonomically designed products, such as scissors, keyboards, and office chairs. The Arthritis Foundation reviews products and gives their Ease of Use designation to those best suited to preserving joints. Among those chosen are wide-grip pens and pencils, an easy-opening coffee container, and a hands-free computer mouse. You may find that some devices are reimbursable by insurance if they are purchased at a pharmacy with a prescription.

There are many choices among the things you regularly use. Wheels, for example, are best for moving things—utility carts and tea wagons. You may find small-wheeled suitcases efficient for storing and moving projects. Wire shopping carts have a multitude of uses.

Choose lightweight alternatives: fiberfill or down rather than wool blankets, a plastic bucket in place of a stoneware crock. The culture has been moving in this direction (compare steamer trunks to canvas luggage), so you will find a lot of choices in this category. Use leverage by choosing long handles and extenders. Buy or make tools with thick handles to open your hand grip. Remember, too, that those around you are resources: I once stood out in the street with a jar of pickles until a jogger came along and kindly opened it for me.

These aids cover best- and worst-case needs, so choose from among them what can be helpful to you. See the Resources section at the back of this book to find aids.

Clothing and getting dressed

The philosopher George Santayana called fashion "innovation without reason and imitation without benefit." You need to choose clothes with reason and benefit—easy to put on and easy to care for. Clothes designed for travel tend to be stylish, wrinkle resistant, or wash and wear. Ironing is stressful to the wrist and time consuming, even if you are the rara avis who likes to do it.

If your fingers are sore, keep closures to the front, substitute Velcro for buttons, or avoid fooling around with fasteners altogether by wearing elasticized waists. Turtlenecks can be trying; my head was once stuck inside a sweater long enough for me to contemplate the patterns of light coming through the weave. Most women don't need to be told to fasten their bras in the front and then reverse them, RA or no; some prefer front-closure bras. A small wire ring on a zipper pull can be helpful. A reaching stick, something like the ones used for picking up litter, can be used to pull up pants or get clothes down from racks. Buttons on sleeves can be sewn on with elasticized thread that will give enough for your hand to slide through easily without unbuttoning.

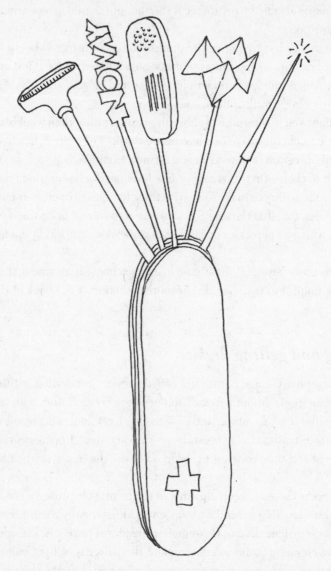

The RA Swiss Army knife, euquipped with a) vacuum for vacuous miracle cures, with no vacuum bag since they are made of air; b) sign for use when tempted to overcommit; c) recorded message: "RA is not the same as OA, etc, not catching, etc."; d) cytokine catcher, works on same principle as e) magic wand that alleviates symptoms when used with ample exercise, rest, medication, and good food.

Shoes and orthotics

> *If high heels were so wonderful, men would still be wear-*
> *ing them.*
>
> —SUE GRAFTON

About 90 percent of people with arthritis eventually have it in their feet and ankles, which are made up of more than a quarter of the bones in the body. As you know by now, every step you take puts multiple times your body weight on your lower extremities. In addition, misalignment of one joint subjects the neighboring structures to increased stress. Because weakening or falling of the **metatarsal**, the ball of the foot, can result from RA, shoes need to be low and provide ample room for your toes.

Which exerts more pressure, an elephant's foot or a high-heeled shoe? A high heel, by more than fifteen times. The American Podiatric Medical Association calls them "biomechanical and orthopedically unsound." The obvious problems are crushed toes and bunions. Researchers at Boston's Spaulding Rehabilitation Hospital found that high heels also shift your weight unnaturally onto your inner knee, increasing torque on the joint near the back of the kneecap and making it susceptible to damage. Chunky high heels proved no better than stilettos. Women are twice as likely as men to develop osteoarthritis of the knee. If you are passionate about your Manolos, you'll need to take some anthropological perspective; there was a time and place where the fragility and helplessness of women was celebrated with bound feet.

Have your shoes fitted later in the day, when there may be more swelling. Running shoes are often orthopedically sound. Many companies make good walking shoes, like Birkenstock and Rockport. (Some lines within brands allow the inner lining to be removed so that your own foot pad can be substituted, like Birkenstock's Footprints.) Zippers or Velcro closures can be handy. You can adapt sneakers with Velcro to replace shoelaces (like the Speed Strap, originally designed for triatheletes).

Cushioned insoles are available from a pharmacy. An arch support will help bear weight. I have much more advanced damage in my feet than you are likely to get; even so, you may want to consider custom-made orthotic inserts. They can take the pressure off your metatarsals and redistribute it across your stabilized arch. Having them has made a great difference for me.

A study of children with juvenile rheumatoid arthritis showed that they did much better with custom orthotics than with over-the-counter inserts.

Somewhere in my saga, before I was correctly diagnosed, I was fitted with toe-straightening contraptions to be worn in bed at night. The only effect they had was to cause my husband's eyes to roll. There are helpful gizmos, however, like long-handled shoehorns, shoelace fasteners, and a device for pulling up socks.

Metatarsal problems can cause the ball of the foot to develop calluses. They can build up and create painful pressure. You can have them removed every few months by a podiatrist or keep a pumice stone at your bath.

In the bathroom

Consider safety and use a rubber bathmat or nonskid strips in the shower, and install grab bars next to the tub. A shower caddy can keep soap and shampoo within reach; there are also wall dispensers. If you have difficulty standing or getting out of the tub, try using a shower bench or a plastic chair so that you can sit while bathing. A removable showerhead with a long hose can be helpful and provides a relaxing massage as well. Perhaps a short wash-and-wear haircut would make a difference.

A bath mitt or two washcloths sewn together can allow you to keep your hand flat while you wash. A sponge with a long, wide handle will reach your back. You can let go of toweling off by slipping into a terrycloth robe and patting yourself dry (but mine takes up half the washing machine). Try a plug for your overflow drain that allows you to fill your tub to a high level for a good soak.

At the bathroom sink: long-handled brush and comb; electric toothbrush and WaterPik; device with a handle that holds dental floss, toothpaste pump (or use the heel of your hand to squeeze the tube). You can enlarge the handles on razors, eyeliner, or mascara by putting a foam rubber hair curler over them.

A friend who has had RA for decades was once stuck on the toilet for hours until her husband came home; she discovered that it is possible to make origami with toilet paper. A conventional toilet seat can be raised by about two inches with a riser, making it easier to stand up if your knees are cranky. When there are long lines at the porta-potty, carry your own; special devices are made for women, but another friend carries a collapsible canvas pet water bowl, which is easily washed and does not have such an obvious use.

Feminine hygiene can get complicated, too. A tampon string can be more easily removed if it is wound around a pencil. When pads are used, a detachable shower hose may be useful for washing.

At work

The theme continues here; make life easier for yourself. Use wheels, reachers to pick things up, thick grips for pens, pencil grips, Fiskars scissors, Peta roller blade cutter, a clamp-on pistol grip for tools such as paint brushes.

Wrist splints are true joint savers. They are available from the drug store, they reverse to adapt to the opposite hand, and are washable; the light-colored ones get dingy fast and never really refresh in the wash, so you may prefer black. Finger splints are useful, too. One friend had hers made out of silver and wears it as jewelry to the university receptions she hosts.

Whatever the name, a laptop does not belong atop the lap, where it distorts your posture. See the first chapter in this section for the biodynamics of working at a desk. Check out a touch-pad device that moves a computer cursor with less strain on your fingers. Inventory your body at regular intervals for tension and maintain a stretching and rest routine.

In the kitchen

Simple cooking does not have to mean lousy food. The closer that fruits and vegetables are to their natural state, the more nutrients they retain, so you save more than your joints when you make dishes with minimal preparation.

Take note of the advantages of planning the week's menu in advance, discussed in Day 6: Living. A Crock Pot allows you to start one pot meals in the morning, when your energy is fresher. I use mine all winter. All summer long I use a solar cooker. In the morning I put the lightweight box on the porch with a pot of any slow-cooking food, say a chicken with a few sprigs of rosemary and some vegetables. By dinnertime it's succulently ready to eat. Solar cooking is versatile; Ruth Reichl, editor of *Gourmet* magazine, extols it.

Avoid lifting heavy pots; try steaming vegetables in frying baskets so that you can lift them out without hefting the pot. Spaghetti cookers have perforated inserts. Or ladle the contents out with a perforated spoon.

If you have the luxury of remodeling a kitchen, a commercial water hose over the stove saves lifting pots of water from sink to stove. Select appliances with levers and buttons that are easy to turn. Some knobs can be replaced with T-shaped handles. I regret not testing the hard-to-open lid of my food processor before I bought it.

Milk cartons make ideal storage for divided portions of leftovers, and you can open them for use as a cutting surface, which allows you to handily move and pour the cut food. Line pans with aluminum foil to save your hands from scrubbing. Use nonstick pans, Silfat sheets, or spray-on cooking oil. Prop a bowl of batter in a pot when you pour it into a baking pan. Stabilize mixing bowls on a rubber mat or damp cloth, or avoid stirring altogether by using a mixer. Work on a stool as much as possible. You can place a bowl or cutting board in a drawer if it is at a more comfortable work height.

For cutting, use your food processor as much as you can for chopping, slicing, or grating. To cut by hand, use an ergonomically designed knife with a curved handle, a chopping knife with single or double blades, or even a round pizza cutter. Oxo now makes a line of kitchen tools with wide handles.

Devices for opening jars range from a round rubber gripper to an under-the-counter device of graduated widths. The rubber grippers are also handy for opening gas caps and folding around handles as grips.

With mitt pot holders, you can lift hot pans with the palms of both hands. I never found this useful, but some people like to pull out hot oven shelves with a bent coat hanger or a dowel with a hook. Other aids are: a can claw; electric can opener; box topper; thick-handled tools like a soap dispenser brush, whisk, ice cream scoop, and peeler.

At home

Let plenty of natural light into your house to brighten your mood. Put full-spectrum bulbs in your lamps. If you can, place a chair outside where you can relax. A lap desk, with a cushion under the surface to hold it, can spare your hands from holding a book up.

Specially designed knobs for lighting fixtures, wall switches, and washing machines are available, as well as lever door handles. Some lamps have a touch device to turn them on or off.

Choose chairs high enough to rise from, or use a lifter seat or chair leg extenders. Locking wheels on furniture make cleaning easier.

If you clean house yourself, as I do, the job is best done in small increments. Keep duplicate sets of cleaning supplies in the areas where they are used. You can clean the bathtub from a stool next to the tub and use a wide, long-handled brush. I use a scrub mitt and do a little each time I take a shower. Try long handles—on a sponge to clean around windows and other hard-to-reach areas, and on your dustpan. Among various other helpful aids are: key turner that provides extended leverage, needle holder, gas cap turner, offset clippers, outside faucet turner.

Laundry is easily carted about in wire shopping carts. I wash a lot of T-shirts for a house full of athletes and put them on hangers to avoid folding them. When it's time to choose, front-loading washers and dryers are easier to deal with. Use a reacher or a backscratcher to pull clothes out of the dryer. If there is no option but to iron, use an adjustable-height ironing board so that you can sit down; consider, though, that training a son to do his own dress shirts would make him a highly desirable mate. Use a smaller container for detergent, unless, like me, you use a huge one with a handled measuring scoop.

Caring for children

Carriers and strollers are now designed to hold infant car seats, making them easier to move. But babies grow, and it becomes increasingly difficult to lift them in and out of a car. You may want to schedule multiple errands when there is care for your child, plan to go with another person, or delegate the trips out. Most clothes for children are designed to be easy to take on and off, but test buttons and snaps to see how you do. Choose Velcro when possible. You can monitor your child's room with an intercom.

Keeping joints warm

You can maintain the heat in your joints with leg warmers, long underwear (silk or one of the new thin fabrics), warm blankets, slipper socks, sweat suit, thermoelastic gloves. Sit with your legs in a sleeping bag to read. To warm up your joints: Put rice or beans in a sock and heat in a microwave about two to three minutes, wrap in a towel; soak sore hands in hot water; use microwave heat wraps; warm hands on a mug filled with a hot drink.

For cold, use an ice pack, ice cubes, gel packs, bag of frozen vegetables.

Using a cane

Sometimes it's wise to put aside pride for pragmatism and use a cane. The length is measured with your arms hanging down at a relaxed angle, with the crease of the wrist determining the height of the cane. For most people, this comes to within an inch of half of their height. Canes come in various strengths according to your weight. Choose as wide a tip as possible, fitted with a rubber end, which can be replaced. Also available is an ice-gripping tip.

Homemade devices

You can build up handles of silverware, brushes, pens, tools, and kitchen utensils with pipe insulation tubing. I just brought some to a friend, and it worked beautifully on crutches and a walker. It is inexpensive and comes in four-foot lengths with openings from ⅜". Simply tape the slit in the tubing closed. You can use foam rubber hair curlers in the same way.

Rubber mesh shelf liner can be used as a pen grip, jar opener, or stabilizer for a mixing bowl. Large rubber bands wound around doorknobs make them easier to grip. A zipper hook can be made from a dowel or the end of wooden spoon and a cup hook. A button hook can be fashioned from a loop of wire duct-taped to a wooden handle. A box slipped into its own cover can serve as a playing card holder. It can be used to hold recipes as well.

You may never need these devices, but then again, they may save you some grief.

IN A SENTENCE:

> Using products and techniques for easing pressure on joints will reduce the risk of damage from RA.

HALF-YEAR MILESTONE

What a difference half a year makes. You have gained perspective on your diagnosis and taken steps to manage it. The specter of rheumatoid arthritis no longer governs your life; you govern your RA. You have learned:

○ HOW IMPORTANT YOUR EMOTIONAL WELL-BEING IS TO YOUR PHYSICAL HEALTH.

○ TO MAKE YOUR EXERCISE PROGRAM A HIGH PRIORITY.

○ TO REPLENISH VITAMIN DEFICIENCIES WITH NUTRITIOUS FOOD, AND LIGHTEN WEIGHT ON JOINTS.

○ TO MAINTAIN A RECORD OF SYMPTOMS AND MEDICAL VISITS AS WELL AS A JOURNAL OF YOUR PROGRESS TOWARD GOALS FOR EXERCISE AND NUTRITION.

○ TO BE AWARE OF BIODYNAMICS THAT CAN AFFECT YOUR JOINTS.

○ TO INTEGRATE SLEEP, REST, AND RELAXATION INTO YOUR DAILY PLAN.

The Immune System and How It Responds in RA

WHY READ fiction? The immune system is more incredible, and, anyway, I couldn't make this stuff up. Apart from the fun, understanding it explains how new drugs are targeted and what researchers are up to.

Focus down to the cellular level. Each of your cells carries all the genes it takes to make another you (except sperm or egg with half). The individual components of the cell are not alive, but the cell is a living sac of chemicals. It communicates in molecules directed by the cell's genes. Receptors on the cell's membrane select signals out of a chemical sea, and, in response, the cell alters its own chemistry to regulate its activity. In this way, the billions of cells that make up the immune system interact in an elegant, mobile community.

Meet the cast of characters—white cells or **leukocytes** (from Greek *leuko*—white), independent single-cell organisms. Not long ago, they were considered a closed system that simply responded to infection. We now know that the immune system is intricately interconnected with the nervous system, which is one good reason that it won't help to stress over remembering all this.

The six types of leukocytes all descend from identical stem cells produced in the bone marrow. Leukocytes make up only about 1 percent of our blood, but they are a powerful minority. They move through the blood stream as well as through the **lymphatic system**. Some form natural barriers in the skin, tears, and saliva. Others have more specialized roles.

Our environment is alive with microscopic creatures. A bacterium can divide two or three times in an hour; at that rate, it can shortly become millions. The leukocytes, like bouncers at the velvet rope, decide who's in and who's out. Inhale someone's sneeze and leukocytes identify and get rid of pathogens that would like nothing better than to eat you alive.

Leukocytes work as a team. The first ones to show up are **neutrophils**, the most common leukocytes. Billions are produced daily in your bone marrow and live about a day. They troll the system for **antigens**—anything they detect as foreign—and function like vacuum cleaners to clean them up.

Roaming leukocytes identify an antigen as anything without a permanent tag that labels it as a "self" cell. This marker is so complex that, except for twins, it is unique to each person. Every leukocyte needs to read that marker accurately every time.

When unmarked cells are detected, neutrophils send out **chemical signals**, bringing other leukocytes on the team into the infected area. They order an increase in fluid, producing inflammation that serves as a barrier to contain the antigens. They summon the next leukocytes to arrive on the scene, the **macrophages**.

Macrophages work like Pac-Man (macrophage means "big eater"), gobbling up each antigen by attaching to its surface, slowing it down and disassembling it. Macrophages in turn send chemical messages to attract the most specialized leukocytes—the **B cells** and the **T cells**.

A macrophage displays a fragment of the digested antigen for identification by the new arrivals. "Helper" T cells stimulate B cells to produce **antibodies**. (Antibodies are proteins that can grab on to matching antigens and dispose of them.) B cells do this by generating **plasma cells**—factories that produce about two thousand specific antibodies per second over a few days. B cells recognize a pathogen that has been encountered before; they simply rev up production of matching antibodies, which then overwhelm the antigen. The task is done without a thought on our part, like predawn garbage collection. Over your lifetime, your B cells may produce as many as ten million different types of antibodies, some created in response to vaccines.

What if the antigen is unknown? B cells tool up to manufacture a new antibody. That can take a few days, allowing the pathogens to party until there are enough antibodies to engulf them. If the same antigen returns, the B cells or their descendents are ready with the pattern on file when the neutrophils put in an order.

B cells, as remarkable as they are, cannot reach an antigen that has penetrated a cell membrane. Who gets the call? Postgrad T cells.

To become a T cell, a new lymphocyte travels from the bone marrow through the blood stream to the **thymus gland** (from which it gets its eponymous T). There it enters a tough school: learn or die. The novice T cell acquires two chemical receptors to detect antigens. These are like locks to keep self cells safe, and a match must be made by both locks before an antigen is destroyed. The T cells are exposed to self cells from the body, such as muscle or cartilage, to test if the locks hold. More than 90 percent of the aspiring T cells do not pass, and they die for their failure. Those who successfully protect self cells go through more selection before taking up duty circulating between the lymph system and the blood.

T cells divide into several different types—for example, those "helper" T cells that prompt the B cells to produce antibodies. But when the "helper" T cells determine that an antigen has penetrated self cell walls, it calls for the only leukocytes that can kill the infected cells—"killer" T cells. Finally, when an infection is overcome, "suppressor" T cells slow the immune response to a stop. It can happen while you are putting on your socks.

I wouldn't believe it possible if it weren't all true. The immune system is so delicate and complex that it is not surprising that it does not function perfectly all the time.

The immune system in RA

We know that the normal immune system is an intricate network of white cells that keeps us healthy. So what's up with ours?

To get some perspective, what's wrong is small compared to what's right. There are about a hundred quadrillion bacterial cells in and on each of us, not to mention other pathogens. That is about ten times the number of cells that comprise us. The legions dining on my detritus as I write and on yours as you read are undaunted, wash as we will. Our immune systems are doing a splendid job keeping us from being consumed. Those of us with RA still recover from cuts, colds, and worse. In RA the immune system works very well indeed.

It is speculated that RA may start with leukocytes (white blood cells) going to work as they are programmed to do by their genes to clean up the usual suspects. Normally, infection is cleared, the large number of leukocytes is reduced to normal, and protective inflammation subsides.

As you have seen, the immune response is complex; the actions of different components have an effect on the actions of others. This is described as the **cascade effect**. We now recognize that in rheumatoid arthritis, the immune system's inflammatory response continues. Like the buckets of water to the sorcerer's apprentice, the leukocytes just keep coming.

In RA, the site of this overresponse is in the membrane that surrounds the entire movable joint, the **synovium**. The first-line leukocytes, the neutrophils, arrive in the synovium to digest microbes and cellular debris that has accumulated in the joint fluid. Perhaps there are more antigens than the neutrophils can handle, or perhaps their chemical message has a hanging molecule, reading "do" instead of "done." They broadcast chemical signals to bring more specialized leukocytes—macrophages, which in turn call B cells and T cells.

These far-reaching chemical messages that turn gene activity on or off are proteins called **cytokines**. At least twenty-four different cytokines may play a role in RA. For example, inflammatory cytokines are released by the macrophages. The mix of cytokine messages determines whether T cells will differentiate into cells that promote or diminish inflammation. In the joints of people with RA, inflammatory T cells are twice as common. Cytokines signal the synovium to swell in weight and volume by twenty to a hundred times. I experienced this phenomenon as a knee as large as a Texas grapefruit and just as bendable.

A wide variety of harmful effects beyond pain and stiffness can be caused by the proliferation of cytokines in RA—anemia, difficulty sleeping, and fatigue. Eventually, unchecked, it can lead to erosion of cartilage and bone, as well as **vasculitis**, inflammatory damage to the lining of the blood vessels.

By some further sorcery, some leukocytes do not heed the controlling signals that cause them to die; they crowd the joints, making immortality less attractive than we'd ever considered.

This is enough but not all. You will recall that B cells produce specific

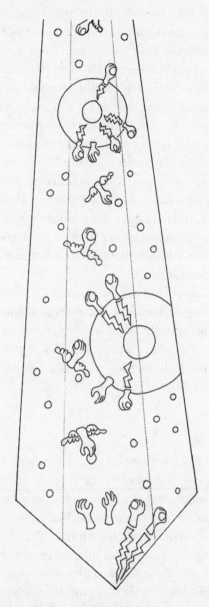

Rheumatologis's Necktie. Design for a painted
silk necktie depicting proliferating cytokines in
RA being grabbed up by molecules of a biologic
drug. Gift to Dr. Ken Sack.

antibodies. People with RA have normally functioning B cells, but some also have B cells that make **autoantibodies**—antibodies that target a person's own antibodies (specifically **IgG**) as foreign. These autoantibodies are called Rheumatoid Factor and are present in 60 to 80 percent of adults with RA. Your diagnosis will involve a test for Rheumatoid Factor.

B cells churn out antibodies that end up in a sticky deposit along the tissue-thin lining of the synovium. It thickens into **pannus**, a deposit that slowly grows from the edges of the joint capsule toward its center, stiffening the joint. As your condition improves, pannus can dissolve.

According to research at Harvard Medical School, as RA progresses over years, the leukocytes continue in a runaway pattern. The chain of events ending in destructive inflammation is no longer triggered by a T cell response to a joint specific autoantigen. Other components of the immune system, like neutrophils, take over in complete autonomy from the T and B cells originally involved at onset.

To sum it up, we know a lot about the onset of RA, but there is a lot we don't know. Welcome to the labyrinth of ambiguity about what's going on in our immune systems with RA. Keep in mind that there is a difference between a labyrinth and a maze. A maze is intended to confuse, a labyrinth to instruct. Much of our path has been mapped, giving us useful patterns, and we are all about finding our way through.

Immunization

Many of us with RA take medications that suppress an overactive immune system. For the most part, we still recover reasonably well from other illness, but the medication could impair the body's ability to ward off serious illness like influenza or pneumonia. For that reason, many physicians recommend a yearly flu shot for people with RA.

Influenza is a highly contagious virus infection easily spread in respiratory droplets from one person to the next. Other respiratory viruses can produce flu-like symptoms, but they are not actually influenza, which is much more severe. Washing your hands is a preventative, but the best protection is vaccination. In some people with compromised immune systems, flu can be very serious, even lethal. Even if you have had the flu, unlike with measles or chicken pox, you do not necessarily have immunity to new strains.

The vaccine contains dead influenza viruses that cannot cause infection. Side effects beyond redness at the injection site are rare, but some people get a mild fever and aching muscles.

The flu shot produced each season contains the three strains of virus thought to be the most prevalent. These strains can change every year, so most people benefit from yearly immunization.

Discuss any vaccinations with your doctor. Sometimes it is recommended that people with RA get vaccinated against a form of pneumonia with Pneumovax. Be aware that some live vaccines should not be taken with particular medications. Keep a record of your immunizations in your medical journal.

IN A SENTENCE:

> *The cascade of responses by the immune cells to protect the body from foreign intrusion is compromised in RA—useful information in understanding how therapies work.*

The Search for Causes

HOW DID we get rheumatoid arthritis? That question is considered by some to be one of the great mysteries in medicine. I visited an undaunted, quick-minded researcher in the quest to discover the answers, Dr. Lindsey Criswell, who heads the Rheumatoid Arthritis Genetics Research Unit at the University of California at San Francisco.

Dr. Criswell is quick to point out that this is not the work of any individual; her team coordinates with others nationwide in a large and ambitious effort to identify the genes responsible for the development of rheumatoid arthritis—NARAC (The North American Rheumatoid Arthritis Consortium). The study, conceived some ten years ago, has performed thousands of genetic tests at a dozen research centers and has come up with evidence of connections between specific genes and RA.

There was no sense of mystery in our conversation. Dr. Criswell's tone conveyed the clear intention that this painstakingly careful research will go on, successfully identifying the genes that determine risk. It was with the satisfied anticipation of a foregone conclusion that she noted that there are more genes to find.

Who gets RA?

About 1 percent of people worldwide have RA, over two million Americans. All ages get it, but most are thirty to fifty at onset. Three-quarters of people with RA are women, with the majority premenopausal when they are diagnosed. There are geographic and ethnic variations. Smoking can predispose to the disease. Stress, too, can influence the immune system. An interplay of elements, both genetic and environmental, appears to be responsible for the disease, as well as for the variations in symptoms from one person to another.

RA is, historically speaking, a new disease. When we read about arthritis found in ancient Egyptian mummies, it is osteoarthritis caused by wear. The earliest evidence of RA is in remains of North American Indians, who today are affected three to five times more than the general population. In contrast, one-tenth as many cases are reported among rural South African blacks and Japanese. Researchers in Japan recently identified a gene that could be diagnostic for RA, but no clear evidence has been found that links it to RA in Caucasians.

A preview of the gene story

Some diseases are known to be caused by specific genes, but most involve a combination of genes and environmental factors. RA is among those with multiple genetic links that are not clearly understood, similar to diabetes or cancer. Susceptibility to RA appears to be **polygenic**, which means it develops under the influence of several genes. Each of these genes alone probably carries only a small risk for autoimmune disease. However, when certain of these genes occur together in the same individual, the risk for developing RA is increased. Furthermore, particular genes not only influence susceptibility but also RA **phenotype** (disease expression) and severity.

To discover where such predisposing genes are located, NARAC identified families in which two or more siblings had RA and, over the last five years, completed genome-wide scans on a thousand sibling pairs. This data has already revealed the locations of at least six different genetic regions involved in susceptibility.

The ultimate goal of this work is identification of specific susceptibility genes. It is the search for a needle in a haystack, but the haystack is now significantly smaller. The next phase of the study focuses on individuals with RA whose parents are both living (trio families). Clues from the previous genome scans will direct closer study in these volunteer trio families.

One cluster of genes involved with immune function has long been known to be involved with RA: the **HLA** (human leukocyte antigen) complex. The study has found the strongest evidence for linkage to RA in one of the genes in that region called HLA-DRB1. (I suppose geneticists don't have the same luxury for creative naming as biologists and astronomers.) Variations of HLA genes can influence how RA develops; people with particular variants are more likely to have severe disease. Two variant HLA genes often result in more severe symptoms. But individuals without specific DRB1 risk variants can still develop RA, and many with these risk variants never get the disease. Dr. Criswell thinks that probably two or more additional genes in the HLA region will also prove to be important.

An important discovery has recently been made by NARAC. A non-HLA gene that is unequivocally a risk factor for the disease has been identified (PTPN22). The gene reduces the deactivation signal to T cells, which functions like taking the air out of the factory whistle, leaving everyone to work obliviously into overtime.

What is especially intriguing about this gene is that it is found in people with several other autoimmune diseases including lupus, type 1 diabetes, and autoimmune thyroid disease. It is not, however, connected to all autoimmune diseases, indicating that there are different pathways leading to various autoimmune diseases. About 25 percent of people with RA were found to have the gene variant.

But 15 percent of people in the general population carry the variant, too, including Dr. Peter Gregersen, the chief NARAC researcher. The discovery that he carries the PTPN22 gene variant came as a surprise, but he considers his risk for getting RA to be low; he understands that it takes more than one gene variant for predisposition to the disease, and he has eliminated other risks like smoking. In fact, he speculates that the gene may strengthen his immune system against infection.

Statistically, if you have one copy of this gene variation, your risk of RA is doubled. If you have two copies (one from each parent), it goes up to four times the risk.

Climbing the family tree

What about our children? They may or may not inherit some or all of our relevant genes, if we have any. If they do, they inherit only a predisposition, not the disease. Mendel, the monk who figured out the principles of heredity, would be scratching his head; RA is not passed on like blue eyes or curly hair.

NARAC hopes to discover how these genes travel in the family tree. Even among those who inherit identified genes, only a minority develop the disease. If one identical twin has RA, the other twin has about a 15 percent chance of having it also. Siblings of people with RA are two to ten times more likely to develop RA themselves over the course of their lifetime—with about 90 percent not getting it.

Other autoimmune diseases, such as lupus, autoimmune thyroid disease, and juvenile diabetes also occur at a higher rate in family members of people with RA. There is a tendency for family members who get RA to have similar disease features, for example in age of onset, positive rheumatoid factor, and development of nodules. Gender certainly plays a role. Men appear to have a phenotype of RA that can involve larger joints like the hips. Premenopausal women are much more likely than men to develop RA, but the numbers level off after age fifty. Three-quarters of pregnant women with RA go into a remission that reverses after they give birth. Women who breastfeed have a lower risk of developing RA; the longer they nurse, the smaller the risk becomes, even decades later.

Still, no sex-linked genes have been identified among the known risk genes. It is speculated that, rather than having different influencing genes, men and women respond differently to the risk genes.

What is the hope?

What value is there in finding the genetic factors in RA? Not a few researchers dedicate their lives to the search, and they are bold enough to use the word "cure." "Understanding the genetic factors in these diseases may allow us not only to decrease disease severity but to interrupt the cycle before it begins," said Dr. Criswell.

In a future that is already in development in the lab, genes can be modulated by substances called small molecule inhibitors, which can change the threshold of a particular immune response. It may be possible for treatment to be influenced by the knowledge that an individual has genetic markers for susceptibility or severity.

The research is still bench science—in the lab, and more academic than commercial. But the work of Dr. Criswell and her colleagues across the country and around the globe brings this future closer every day. The technology to do this is advancing rapidly. In the last five years, the ability to examine genetic variations in the lab is one hundred times faster.

Our genes are part of the puzzle. For now, they are what we cannot change. Other influences also contribute to our predisposition to the disease and to the course it takes, and that is where we can create change.

Environmental influences

Little has been known about other causes of RA—broadly defined as environmental factors. It was a field littered with myth: arthritis is caused by cold, damp weather; tomatoes, potatoes; knuckle cracking. The influence of genetic factors is lower in RA than in some other autoimmune diseases, leaving a lot of possibility for other contributing causes. Dr. Criswell has set about mapping that territory at the crossroads of nature and nurture.

A huge body of data gathered over eleven years from half of the middle-aged women in the state of Iowa (**The Iowa Women's Health Study**) yielded a wealth of information available to Dr. Criswell and her colleagues. They identified the women who later developed RA and evaluated their exposures to potential environmental risk factors. The exposure information is especially valuable because it was determined before RA diagnosis. Memory tends to select events to match an outcome; this data has no "recall bias," making it more dependable.

The Iowa study found no relation between the onset of RA and physical characteristics such as height, weight, body mass index, leisure time physical activity, or alcohol use. (That is not to say that most of these factors do not affect the progress of the disease.)

No butts about it

Among the women in the study, smoking led to an approximately twofold increased risk of RA. In a separate study of both men and women, researchers in Sweden examined the contributions of two specific risk factors: a particular HLA gene and cigarette smoking. They found that for people who had the gene but had who never smoked, the increased risk for RA was about triple. For current cigarette smokers without the gene, the risk factor increased almost as much. For current smokers with the gene, however, the risk increased by nearly sixteen times over that of nonsmokers without the same genetic profile. The conclusion is that smoking alone increases the risk of RA, and it significantly increases the risk among people with a genetic predisposition for the disease.

Cigarette smoke appears to increase levels of rheumatoid factor (RF), the autoantibody active in RA. "Cigarette smoking is the strongest environmental risk factor identified to date for rheumatoid arthritis," says Dr. Elizabeth Karlson of Harvard. The report from the Iowa study concluded that RA should be added to the list of smoking-related diseases.

It is thought that other environmental triggers could include prolonged infection and exposure to toxins such as CO_2, silica, or asbestos. Studies in China and Africa found strikingly higher rates of RA among people with similar genetic backgrounds living in urban areas. It is speculated that some combination of pollution, exposure to disease, and stress may contribute.

Coffee, not guilty as charged

Coffee, once thought to be a risk factor, was exonerated by the Iowa study. Tea also was found not to contribute; it may possibly even lower risk. Decaffeinated coffee, however, at more than four cups a day, appeared to increase disease risk—perhaps due to chemicals previously used in processing. It was confirmed that coffee or tea did not increase the risk of developing RA in another study, the Nurses' Health Study, where eighty-three thousand women completed questionnaires every four years over an eighteen-year period. That study did not confirm the association of decaffeinated coffee with RA; however it did confirm that smoking is associated with an increased risk of RA.

Stress as a factor

Psychoneuroimmunolgy is a branch of medicine that examines the relationship between the mind, the nervous system, and the immune system.

Although the immune system was once thought to be autonomous, we now know know that it is closely linked with the nervous system and the endocrine system. Many different chemicals come through nerves down the spinal cord from the brain that can increase or decrease the activity of leukocytes.

There is a body of evidence that has linked stressful experiences or events with altered immune system functioning, including overactivation of the immune system. Stress can affect the degree to which lymphocytes multiply, the activity of "killer" T cells, and the proliferation of antibodies (particularly IgA).

Some researchers suspect that rheumatoid arthritis is triggered by an infection—possibly a viral or bacterial—in people with an inherited susceptibility.

Moving on

As we each try to understand our individual experience with RA, the contributing causes appear as pieces of a complex and incomplete puzzle. The genetic component varies. There could be a triggering infection, but that's not yet clear. Other environmental conditions like smoking are clearly connected for many but not all. Stress contributes, but to what degree we don't know. Gender must figure in, but both sexes get RA.

There is something liberating in putting these scientific questions into the hands of researchers like Dr. Criswell, setting aside what we cannot know for sure, and taking on our task of managing the disease.

IN A SENTENCE:

> *Genes can predispose a person for RA, as can environmental factors such as smoking, but they are not found in all people who have RA.*

Complications of RA

Life span and heart disease

The road forks when you come to RA. You can become healthier than you have ever been in your life by managing the disease. The other choice, ignoring it, is a dangerous one that can start chains of events linked to progressively unfortunate complications. This chapter is about the road not taken.

Statistically, life expectancy for people with RA is compromised, but current numbers are based on people who did not have access to the drugs and information that you now have to manage it. Also, every individual with RA responds differently, and the progress of the disease cannot be predicted with certainty.

The National Institute of Arthritis and Musculoskeletal and Skin Diseases (NIAMS), with scientists at the Stanford University School of Medicine, found that the average disability levels for people with RA declined over twenty years from 1977 by 40 percent, a rate of about 2 percent a year. The time frame for this study corresponds to the period during which the use of the drug methotrexate became standard, treatment became more aggressive, and the evaluation of exercise changed. Since the end of that study, the biologic drugs have been introduced, and they offer hope of even further reductions in disability.

Still, I would be remiss not to tell you that several epidemiology studies have shown a significantly higher rate of cardiovascular disease and related deaths among people with RA. In a Mayo Clinic study it was determined that markers of systemic inflammation are associated with a significantly increased risk for cardiovascular death. They found the odds of developing congestive heart failure, or a weakening of the heart's ability to pump blood, was double in RA patients. Scientist at Brigham and Women's Hospital in Boston concluded from the large Nurses' Health Study of women that levels of several inflammatory biomarkers linked to heart disease were significantly elevated in those with RA. These studies and others show that systemic inflammation in RA is dangerously linked to heart disease.

Furthermore, the Mayo Clinic group reported that the RA patients were less likely to report symptoms of angina. Another study found RA patients lacking in important aspects of primary care. Keep up appointments with your general practitioner, who will follow your risk for dangers that can accompany RA, and forgive me for repeating this reminder.

Stress is a factor

As you know well, having a chronic disease can be stressful. Stress increases blood pressure and constricts blood vessels, both cardiovascular concerns, and stress can also pump up levels of **cholesterol**, **triglycerides**, and **homocysteine**—all indicators of heart disease.

Researchers at the University of California at San Francisco found that high stress can affect the way that chromosomes divide, eventually causing weakened muscles, deterioration of vision and hearing, and mental decline.

Sleep disturbance, which can be attributed to stress, is reported by nearly three-quarters of people with arthritis. Sleep deprivation leads to a cycle, creating more stress and loss of sleep, and interfering with the brain's ability to modulate pain.

Fatigue can lead to loss of activity and weight gain, both of which have a negative effect on the joints.

Weight gain

Excess cortisol, produced from inflammation, directs fat to build around the abdomen. It is a type of fat that secretes inflammatory chemicals, worsening inflammation in yet another downward cycle.

Diabetes

The same inflammatory chemicals associated with RA can block insulin receptors. This condition of insulin resistance can progress to **type 2 diabetes**.

Eyes and mouth

Some people with RA have an inflammation of the whites of the eye, called **scleritis**. Dry, scratchy, irritated eyes need to be moistened; if left untreated, the condition can lead to further complications.

More serious is Sjögren's syndrome, an autoimmune condition of the moisture-producing glands, which can be diagnosed by a rheumatologist. This condition is found in more than 50 percent of patients with high levels of rheumatoid factor, 90 percent of them women. The resulting dryness in the eyes, nose, mouth, and vagina requires lubrication and in some cases medication. Taste is affected, and the eyes can feel sore. It is sometimes accompanied by **uveitis**, inflammation of the colored parts of the eye.

Decay-causing bacteria are a hundred times more numerous in people with Sjögren's. Normally, at least forty proteins and minerals in saliva protect your mouth and prevent infection. All the nutrients necessary for healthy tooth enamel—calcium, phosphate, fluoride—come from saliva. People with Sjögren's have more plaque, more decayed, filled, or missing teeth, and more bone loss at the roots of the teeth.

Fatigue is another prominent symptom in primary Sjögren's, a disease that presents in varying degrees.

Care of the eyes and teeth are important concerns. Brush and floss regularly, have regular dental exams, as well as daily fluoride treatments. Chewing xylitol gum can help maintain moisture. Use eye drops to supplement your natural tears to soothe, moisturize, and protect your eyes. Dozens of over-the-counter products are available, but first get the advice of a specialist. Avoid products with active ingredients that end in "zoline." Those ingredients are vasoconstrictors designed to reduce redness and should not be used for more than a few days. The film covering the eyes is complicated; an ophthalmologist can tell you if there is an imbalance in any part—the inner layer of proteins, the watery middle layer, or the top oily layer. Then she will recommend the appropriate drops or lubricant. If your eyes are dry and you use eye makeup, use hypoallergenic brands.

It is helpful to set up a humidifier, take frequent breaks from the computer, sip water throughout the day, and remove contacts from time to time. Smoking won't help; it has been linked to eye problems. Avoid caffeine, as it is a diuretic, which means that it causes your body to lose water.

Chest and lungs

Lung problems in RA, a result of the inflammatory process, involve the pleural lining of the lungs. I spoke with a man with RA who had had such inflammation drained four times in thirty years. Again, he did not have access to the regimen that you will use to manage your RA.

Obviously, you should avoid cigarette smoking.

Bones

Measures of bone mineral density of patients with low to moderately active RA show a relationship between the severity of the disease and the risk of bone loss. Stress fractures are a significant risk in active RA. Past steroid use, especially at high doses, adds to the risk. A Norwegian study found a doubled risk of vertebral deformities in RA and a substantially increased risk of hip fractures. In view of the biological consequences of inflammation and longtime steroid use, the researchers conclude that careful control of disease activity benefits the skeleton.

Joint replacement

To understand why arthritis accounts for the majority of joint replacement surgeries, look at sets of joint X-rays taken over a seven-year period at the Web site of the European League Against Rheumatism (www.EULAR.org; go to Working Party in Imaging in Rheumatology, then click on Quantitative

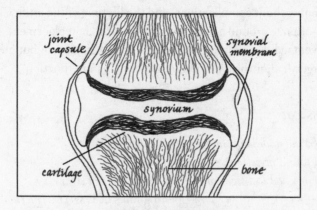

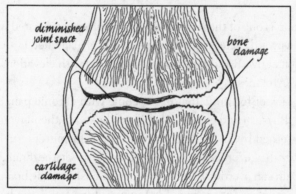

Healthy joint capsule, above, with plenty of space
between the bones taken up with the synovium filled
with synovial fluid. Below, joint capsule with prolonged active rheumatoid arthritis. The joint space is
diminished, cartilage and bone disintegrated.

analysis of radiological progression of rheumatoid arthritis). You will see how
quickly the erosion of cartilage and bone can advance if unchecked.

When normal daily activities become impossible, joint replacement,
the surgical replacement of a joint with an artificial prosthesis, is the last
resort. It is typically done when there is no more cartilage and bone grinds
on bone, causing increasingly unbearable pain. Since the first joint replacement, a hip in 1969, replacements of the knee, hip, and shoulder have been
done frequently. Although joint replacements have a high rate of success,

they are not without complications, and the lifetime of the artificial joint is limited—often to around a decade. Elbow and ankle replacements are still being developed. Small joints of the feet are not replaced, but are fused. Hand surgery can involve tendon transfers to restore function.

Depression

> In the middle of the journey of our life
> I found myself lost in a dark wood
> For I had lost sight of the path that does not stray.
> —opening lines of DANTE's Inferno

Depression is one of the most frequent symptoms associated with RA—part of a downward cycle fueled by pain, which is magnified by depression. Even without active RA, depression is associated with elevations in proinflammatory cytokines.

It is not lack of fortitude that puts people with chronic pain at risk for depression. Physical and emotional pain are linked in the nervous system; both are governed by the same chemical neurotransmitters, such as serotonin, and both are processed in the same parts of the brain. Chronic stress and pain can override normal circuitry, intensifying the brain's distress signals. The subsequent feeling of being out of control is the hallmark of depression.

Attitudes toward depression

Our family has been close to a dear person who has suffered and recovered from depression. I speak frankly here: there is nothing deep, romantic, creative, insightful, or worthwhile about depression. It does not bring artistic insight or literary sensitivity. It is a serious disorder that disrupts families, careers, and aspirations. It can cause brain and nerve cell atrophy. It can be progressive, causing damage to the heart, endocrine glands, and bones.

We all sing the blues from time to time. We suffer loss and worry through change. That is not the same as the pervasive, persistent, empty hopelessness that is depression. It requires treatment. For those of us with RA treading the edge of that abyss, managing our disease helps us to avoid falling in.

Symptoms of depression

It is not easy to recognize depression in yourself. It creeps in by degrees, one day expressed in a sharp word, the next in an indecisive lack of direction. The degrees are indistinguishable from normal fluctuations in mood until they begin to add up: a prolonged feeling of unhappiness, difficulty sleeping, loss of interest in friends, confusion, low self-confidence, a change in eating habits, a feeling of helplessness, carelessness, anger, listlessness, difficulty concentrating, suicidal thoughts.

Treatment

The stigma against treating the brain as an organ of the body still lingers, and the belief that depression requires no more than a stiff upper lip still keeps some sufferers from the rehabilitation they deserve. If you are experiencing symptoms of depression, there are things you can do. Even though you may not feel up to doing any of them, depression feeds on itself, and you need to break the cycle:

Get help. Psychotherapy helps you recognize thoughts and behaviors that trigger stress. Your therapist may recommend a temporary course of medication. Join a support group where you can find a phone buddy. Get professional help immediately if your have suicidal thoughts. The national suicide hot line is 800-784-2433.

Review your program. Report your psychological symptoms to your doctor and assess your medications.

Continue your RA management program. It includes treating your pain with mind-body techniques and, if you choose, medication; exercise, the best natural antidepressant; journaling your thoughts and particularly your pain and mood.

Spruce up. Bathe and dress with care.

Do what you do. Continue your daily routine, even when you are not in the mood.

Moderate alcohol. Alcohol is a depressant, so limit your intake.

Seek out a supportive environment. Stay in touch with compassionate friends and skip unpleasant obligations.

Don't run away. It is said that wherever you go, there you are. It won't be better somewhere else without working through problems first.

Light up your life. Let natural light into your home, use full-spectrum bulbs, and spend as much time outside as you can.

Avoiding complications

The good news here is that we know enough to navigate these shoals. Unless you ignore RA, you do not need to suffer these complications. By following a careful program, you can manage a long and healthy life.

IN A SENTENCE:

> *Untreated RA can result in serious physical and emotional complications—strong motivation to manage the disease well.*

Intimacy, Pregnancy, and Menopause

Intimacy

Arthritis can affect sexual feelings, with aching joints and fatigue proposing the hottest act to be the evening bath. Medications for RA can interfere with sexual functioning as well. One friend with RA called sex "the last thing on my mind for years." It is not the disease that causes a lack of desire, but the physical and emotional stress. Once you experience problems, you may feel anxious or depressed, which can further subdue your sexual feelings.

Let me count the ways that sex can enhance your life—fun, love, health. Sexual activity is correlated with longevity; one New York cardiologist recommends that his patients have sex four times a week for half an hour. Sex releases into the bloodstream endorphins, natural painkillers that also serve to diminish depression. So if you just don't feel like it, perhaps it depends more on what *it* is. Consider that when we are feeling our worst, massage is a pleasure, and being held with love lifts the spirit if nothing else; sex is not only about intercourse. Or even having a partner.

Dr. Jackson Rainer, a psychologist who specializes in treating couples dealing with chronic illness, suggests that the definition of sexuality be broadened to "an energy that is healing, warming, and operates more outside the genitals than in one specific place on the body."

If you have a partner, find a time to talk. It is not uncommon for people to have had a longtime sexual relationship without ever speaking about it. Although the cultural taboo seems to have been lifted in films and books, many people find it difficult or embarrassing to discuss sex privately. Clear communication can dissolve misunderstandings that may have been created by the changes in your health. Dr. Rainer says his favorite four-letter word for intercourse is "talk."

For example, your partner may be afraid of hurting you, and you may have misinterpreted reticence for rejection. You may feel less desirable—perhaps your own feelings about your body with RA and not your partner's. Or you may be hesitant to suggest sensual play that would be comfortable for you. You need to tell your partner what is difficult and what gives you pleasure. Some couples discover that this frankness brings a new sense of intimacy.

Remember together what you did to please each other when you first met. I once wrote small notes to my husband, poems or drawings, but those endearments were lost amidst midnight baby feedings and school lunches as we made our lives together. One therapist has couples make notes of some things that would please them and exchange the lists, reminding them to do something for their mates every so often.

Dr. Rainer suggests an exercise called sensate focusing, a way for each partner to learn about the other's body. In the quiet seclusion of a comfortable bed, one partner slowly touches the other, asking how each move feels and how it could feel better as he explores. It may be helpful to use the same pain scale of one to ten that your doctor uses to communicate your level of comfort. The only rule is that your partner not touch the genitals, since the goal is not orgasm but learning what Dr. Rainer calls a language of touch. This is not my rule, and you don't need to tell me how this assignment works out.

You may do well to plan your lovemaking in advance. If it seems strained, remember the pleasure of anticipating a date. Set the scene with music if you like and low light. Experiment. If you are bushed at night and creaky in the morning, try a noon tryst, which might have the added spice of feeling a little illicit. Perhaps a hot shower will soothe your joints and be a nice place to play. Try new positions to see what feels best, and use whatever physical and emotional stimulation you both enjoy, like oils to enhance massage. Some suggest fantasy, and others find that simply paying attention to the moment gives them a sense of the body and psyche as one.

Spontaneously touch as much as you can during times that you are together. Curl up side by side on the couch, hold hands, enjoy each other's presence.

Be open with your doctor, although it may take some effort. Some medications can have an effect, both positive and negative, so it is important to discuss sex with your health professionals—although fewer than one in five people do. Antidepressants, glucocorticoids (prednisone), muscle relaxants, and other drugs can put a damper on your sex drive. Don't assume that your choice is between effective medication and a satisfying love life. Discuss the option of adjusting your dosage or changing drugs. You or your partner may be afraid that having sex will set off a flare; au contraire, it can be life enhancing. You may need to protect your joints during lovemaking, changing positions and using pillows for support. A woman with dry eyes and mouth from RA can have problems with vaginal lubrication, which can be caused by antidepressants or menopause as well. Over-the-counter lubricants can help. Yeast infections in women can cause irritation, and they require treatment. For a man, there are changes with aging. For both sexes, it takes increasingly longer to climax, so a sexual relationship evolves even without RA; taking your time can make it better, as the song goes about the man with the slow hand. The quality of intimacy need not decline. It is not about kung fu prowess; sex can be shown in a symphony of expression—from caring to passion. It is said that the greatest sex organ is the mind.

The diet and exercise you maintain to manage your RA will also enhance your love life by increasing your energy and decreasing your pain. Sometimes sex can be a gift to your partner that you give when you don't quite feel like it. Then again, after you start, you can change your mind and make it your gift, too.

Getting pregnant

The good news is the wonderful and puzzling fact that three out of four women with RA go into remission during pregnancy. The bad news is that there is no way to know who is the one in four who will not, and none of the medications used in the treatment of arthritis is absolutely safe during pregnancy.

Pregnancy in women with RA is not rare. The pregnancies appear to be relatively normal, with no increase in the rate of cesarean delivery. RA does not seem to decrease fertility, with the exception of severe flares in some individuals. It appears that RA does not harm the fetus, although there are not enough studies to establish a firm conclusion. Not surprisingly, married women with RA have smaller families compared to women who do not have RA. Most women dealing with a chronic disease would think twice before adding the physical and psychological impact of having a child.

Pregnancy needs to be planned, and in some cases quite well in advance. Preconception counseling with your doctor is widely urged. Use contraception while on most DMARDs. Many of these drugs have a prolonged half-life, making it necessary to discontinue them several months before a planned conception—for men as well as women. The potential use of medications during pregnancy needs to be made with a careful assessment of the risks involved.

No markers or indicators have been found to determine which women will not experience relief of symptoms during pregnancy. Although the presence of rheumatoid factor can be an indicator of severity of disease, neither RF, nor age, nor disease duration, nor severity indicates the course of the disease during pregnancy. In some cases, RA intensifies in pregnancy, although it does not tend to involve more joints. Hence, the decision to use medications should be made after careful assessment of the risks and benefits in consultation with your doctor.

Most patients whose RA subsides experience a decrease in the number of joints involved and degree of pain starting with the first trimester. In others, the improvement begins in the second or third trimester. About 16 percent go into remission. Typically, symptoms return during the postpartum period, when there may be a flare. A woman's experience with RA during pregnancy has not been shown to affect the long-term course of the disease. Those who have diminished disease activity during one pregnancy are more likely to have the same experience during subsequent pregnancies.

During pregnancy

During pregnancy, your obstetrician and rheumatologist will need to be in contact. Drugs that you do choose to take during pregnancy need to be closely monitored. Conditions commonly occurring during pregnancy, like morning sickness, can prevent absorption of medications.

Routine obstetrical care includes blood work to check for anemia, particularly important because it is a symptom known to accompany RA. Some pregnancy symptoms can be mistaken for RA symptoms, like swelling of the feet and back pain. It is difficult to measure RA disease activity during pregnancy because the erythrocyte sedimentation rate, sed rate (see Day 5), cannot be used, since pregnancy alters normal values. In general, drug-free pain control during pregnancy is preferable—exercise, mind-body practices, splinting, hot or cold packs.

For pregnant women with RA, sleep needs to be guarded like a treasure. Hormones wake pregnant women up at night, and more than three-quarters of women report that they make frequent trips to the bathroom during the night or wake up in discomfort. Lack of sleep or chronically disrupted REM sleep can promote an appetite-stimulating hormone, as well as slow the production of an appetite-suppressing hormone. The result can be additional stress on the joints from weight in excess of the gain that comes with pregnancy. Fatigue and weight gain can make exercise less likely, leading to pain and depression. Your doctor needs to be attentive following delivery because some women have flares during the postpartum period.

Breastfeeding

It is not clear why, but women who breastfeed have a lower risk of developing RA. The longer they nurse, according to the Iowa Study, the smaller the risk becomes, even decades later. (See Month 8 for a description of the study.)

But in women who have developed RA, there is some evidence that links breastfeeding with postpartum flares. Once again, numerous pharmaceuticals taken by the mother are secreted in milk, and the desire to breastfeed must be balanced with the possible return of RA symptoms.

Theories about RA in pregnancy

Why do so many women with RA go into remission during pregnancy? Ah, that is a question that many researchers would like to answer. Various theories have been proposed, but no single observation explains the improvement entirely. Multiple factors are probably responsible.

No sex-linked genes have been identified among the known risk genes for RA, so it is thought that men and women may respond differently to the same risk genes. (See Month 8, genetics.)

Pregnancy results in an altered immune state to insure that the fetus is not rejected as foreign. Hormonal changes—increased cortisol, estrogen, and progestin—prompt the multiplication of regulatory T cells. There are two kinds of immunity-regulating T cells, one of which promotes and the other of which decreases inflammation. In RA, there is an overabundance of the first type. (See Month 7.) During pregnancy the number of the second type of cells, called helper T cell (Th2), expands to decrease immune activity in order to prevent the rejection of the fetus. It also protects the joints of the mother.

Women whose RA improved during pregnancy were more likely to have an HLA (human leukocyte antigen) disparity with their fetus. HLA are markers on each of your cells that allow your body to differentiate between self and foreign cells. There are over a hundred HLAs, and in women who had a mismatched antigen with their fetus (especially an antigen called HLA DQ), RA subsided. The body appears to hold back the immune response in the presence of the fetus's foreign cells.

Interestingly, the same mechanism in blood transfusion appears to have had a positive effect for some, as reported in the Iowa study. (See Month 8.) It was found that some RA patients, particularly those who were RF positive, got an immunomodulatory effect that lasted years from a transfusion. The odds of improvement rely on the donor and recipient having at least one particular HLA antigen in common and a mismatch for the other one—a situation that mimics the immunologic mechanism active in pregnancy.

Function of neutrophils, other immunity-regulating white blood cells, also decreases in pregnancy.

Postpartum flares have several causes: decreased anti-inflammatory steroid levels, increased inflammatory hormones, and diminished levels of helper T cells in proportion to inflammation-causing T cells.

It is hoped that an understanding of how RA abates in pregnancy will allow the same pathways to be followed in order to mimic the effect on the cells of people who are not pregnant.

Deciding to have a baby

The decision to have a baby is a life-changing one. The possibility of a brief respite from RA is, of course, not a reason to become pregnant. On the other hand, any consideration of passing RA on to your child need not be a factor in your decision. (See Month 8 on genetic inheritance.) We know that there is a genetic predisposition for RA and other autoimmune diseases, but you may not have these genes; if you do, the chance of your baby inheriting them is small, and the chance that she will develop the disease is even smaller.

More germane are considerations of your health as caregiver to a baby, which requires a lot of energy, lack of sleep, and porting the weight of a child around on your already taxed joints. When you plan for a baby, make plans for yourself as well.

Menopause

The remission of RA in pregnancy, with waxing hormonal levels, is but a memory at menopause, when hormones wane, and, for some women, joints ache.

A study in the Netherlands examined age, sex, and women's hormonal levels in patients with RA. Disease activity was not significantly different in male and female patients until women became postmenopausal. At that time, the disease was found to be much more active in those women than in women who had not gone through menopause and than men of the same age. Postmenopausal women also had more joint damage than premenopausal women, possibly because of decreased bone density.

As we have seen with pregnancy, hormones such as estrogen influence immune response. But studies have not found that estrogen replacement therapy protects women against RA. Other hormones may play a role, like progesterone, which rises in pregnancy and declines in menopause.

Other symptoms of menopause can complicate RA management. Hot flashes can interrupt sleep, causing the cascading problems that follow. Weight gain is typical, but it comes from lack of exercise, not from hormonal change.

My grandmother called menopause "the change." You have now a blueprint to make it a change for the better.

IN A SENTENCE:

> *Preparing for the possible influences of RA on intimacy, pregnancy, and menopause will help you enjoy these elements of a well-lived life.*

Organizing Living, Travel, Holidays, and Entertaining

Organizing resources

With RA, we gain a lot by giving up a few things. A helter-skelter life is near the top of the list of what we can do without. With the same blindness with which the unattended disease wanders into mischief, it falls into lockstep behind a healthy routine. Everything we touch and do is a prop or a set for us to lead the dance with RA.

The goal here is not for you to transform yourself into an obsessive-compulsive person, but to use organization of your thoughts, acts, and possessions to relieve chronic stress that exacerbates RA. Lifestyle changes take effort and concentration. They come about slowly, sometimes too slowly for our patience. It takes a leap of faith. That being the case, it is best for you to organize your thoughts first.

Ways of organizing thought

Meditation is a primary tool for organizing the mind. It sweeps clean loose chatter, bags it up, and sets it out for garbage collection—leaving important ideas clear. It sets a reflective rather than a reactive tone. You may benefit the most from a practice of sitting meditation, or you may prefer moving meditation like yoga, tai chi, or even walking. (See Month 5.)

Some habits of mind are a small investment for a large return. Allow time to organize your workspace at the end of the day and prepare your agenda for the next one. This is the trick of the primitive hunter and the modern elite athlete, going through the motions, submitting them in effect to the unconscious, so that when the time comes to act, you move with fluidity of purpose. It doesn't mean, of course, that you can't change your plans, but it gives you a template that you can submit to REM sleep for approval, a list you don't have to keep inventing as you tire in the afternoon.

A behavior modification expert from Stanford University, using an elementary school as a lab, explained to me that it takes many, even hundreds of, repeated internal reminders to form a habit. Following his advice, I have come to deposit my car keys routinely in the same place without a second thought.

Organizing things

A cluttered mind and a cluttered environment feed on one another. Everywhere there are things—things whining, admonishing, grumbling, reminding us that they need attention in one way or another. The cacophony can snarl your day. Many hoarders, random collectors, keepers of things-I-might-need-someday can trace their roots back to the teachings of the Depression generation, or earlier generations, who experienced very real want. Others of us just never got around to going through the closets as new things got jammed in like geologic layers. We sort through a lot of things with this diagnosis—ways of thinking of ourselves and conducting our lives. There is much to get rid of to make room for a new life, and unnecessary nuisance is a good place to start.

If you are attached to your clutter, you may want the eye of someone more objective to help you. The morning may find you less nostalgic. Set about the task in small increments, a shelf, drawer or quarter of a room at a time.

A good trick is to search for useful things to keep rather than getting rid of junk. I met a professional organizer who takes a spiritual point of view; she feels that she is the custodian, the steward, of her possessions, so she sees her second pair of blue slacks as more than her due—something that can be better used by someone else.

Whatever your tactic, decide to decide. Go for it, chanting "Simplify!" as you sort. Set out boxes or bags for various destinations—donations, recycling, garbage, and things you can't quite bring yourself to part with. Adieu, adieu, parting is such sweet sorrow; goodbye to the tennis racquet and spike heels. Have some fun with shedding the old life.

Many local charities will pick up your donation boxes. Seal up the questionables and label the box with a get-rid-of-by date a year hence. If you haven't wakened in the night with a desire for something in there, then, those who know about such things tell us to pass the box on without opening it.

Consider that your need to simplify will trump any obligation to sentiment. Get rid of unwanted gifts and keep the good wishes they were meant to convey. Keep the things that lift your spirits.

Sort into categories that suit you—things that are the most used, easiest to handle. Arrange categories in the way you are most likely to use them, for example, ingredients you would use only for Chinese cooking together rather than being sorted by condiments, noodles, canned goods; separate summer and winter socks since they are used at different times.

Rearrange your house so that things have a place. Put bills into a file or napkin holder by due date, along with their return envelopes, and throw out the ads. Put tax receipts into categorized folders (income, donations, medical deductible). Put your clothes away at night; hooks are handy for nightclothes. If you have an early morning, put out your clothes the night before.

Keep things where you use them, duplicating cleaning supplies at various locations so you don't have to cart them around. A closed basket in our dining nook holds scissors, pens, scratch paper, and tissues.

I asked one professional organizer if she could add a word of advice; her response was "containerize." Use bins, organizers, pull-out shelves, turntables. Sort out-of-season storage into boxes—clear plastic so that you can scan a shelf quickly. Label everything. To avoid rummaging through utensil or tool drawers, use dividers. Translucent containers for the refrigerator will eliminate mystery flora in forgotten meals stored in old yogurt cartons. Pegboards make tools or household items easily accessible, and bulletin boards with clips can hold family messages. For the inevitable odd pieces, have a UFO box, unidentified found objects, which, for some silly reason, we dump out on the table at New Year's, and, when no one claims the contents, we ceremoniously throw it all away.

Organizing time

Once you establish a schedule, it will gain momentum. You'll need a specific time to exercise, to do your mind-body work, to enjoy friends. Do your best to stick with the schedule, even if you don't feel like it, until it takes on a life of its own. Choose a day of the week for medical and other appointments so you can plan to make other stops when you are out. Plot errands in one area, the furthest one first. Call ahead to avoid a wild goose chase.

If you have a choice, time trips to avoid traffic and lines. Both can be avoided by shopping online.

Consider that time allotted to a job can be nil. Ask yourself if the task is any more necessary than the clutter you just put out on the curb for pickup. If it needs to be done, perhaps it can be delegated or simplified. Time invested up front can save considerable time in the process of a job. Think through the steps involved and how to organize them efficiently. Assembling all you need for a task before you begin will save you time; professional chefs work this way and call it *mis en place*. Use time-savers like return labels for correspondence. Break a job down so that you can pace yourself, starting well before the deadline and planning for rest. Deadlines by nature give us a reason to rush and can be stressful. (To keep our work expectations in perspective, Americans work nine weeks more per year on average than their counterparts in Western Europe.)

Distributing big tasks, like keeping house or maintaining a garden, over time can make them doable. Create a schedule, listing tasks to be done on specific days of the week, with heavy work spread out over the month, to be completed on days when you are feeling better. Some things can be done in very small increments: keeping the house picked up can be ongoing as you pass from room to room, depositing things in a basket on the stairs for example; a bucket with a weeding tool can await a daily quota of a dozen weeds or so. A number of organizing books and Web sites are full of good ideas; www.flylady.net has suggestions on housework.

Organizing RA records and medications

Write notes in your medical records promptly and make them brief. (See Month 2.) Keep your medications where you take them, in the kitchen or where you have meals. Separating medications into weekly pillboxes by the day will spare you time and your fingers from repeatedly twisting the bottles open, and the absence of the pills will show that you have taken them. Medications that need to be kept cold are best not kept in the refrigerator door, where temperature fluctuates. Schedule injections for a time of day when clothing will allow you access to your thighs and abdomen, and store alcohol swabs either near where you usually do your injection or with the medication.

Travel/flying

Planning ahead can make the difference between an enjoyable trip and a vacation you have to take a vacation from. Choose a destination to suit your situation.

In any case, pack lightly—half of what you might need—and rinse things out as you go. Use luggage on wheels, and limit your carry-on to a shoulder bag.

If you are flying and have a choice, travel during lighter traffic hours, so that you do not have to wait in line to go through security. If you have metal in your body that would set off the detector, it helps to let security know before you walk through. It's just as well to avoid dressing with metal belt buckles and hair clips that will have to be undone and redone. Notice that the new air passenger chic is sweat pants and flip flops.

Notify the airline of any special needs. Book nonstop flights when you can. If you need to make a connecting flight, a concourse can be half a mile long; you can request cart transport ahead of time. Don't hesitate to ask to preboard if standing is a problem. An aisle or bulkhead seat will give you space to stretch your legs and do range-of-motion exercises. If your medication needs to be refrigerated, mention it to the flight attendant as you board. Pillows and blankets are often no longer available, so pack an inflatable pillow and a warm jacket, since the cabin tends to be cool. If the flight provides food, you can order a special meal or pack something nutritious. Remember to bring water, as the recirculated air in the cabin can be drying.

Driving

Plan a car trip with frequent stops so that you can stretch. Pack medications in the car rather than the trunk, where they would be exposed to more extreme temperatures. If you are renting a car, check ahead for features that will make it easier for you to drive, such as cruise control, a tiltable steering wheel, wide-angled mirrors, and adjustable headrests. Pack a key turner for the ignition if you need it, and a cushion for resting.

A portable restroom system for women, The Freshette Director, allows them to urinate discreetly, standing, sitting, or in bed. As has been mentioned, a collapsible fabric water bowl made for dogs works as well.

Medications

Pack snacks and a water bottle so that you can take your medications on time when you travel. Set a wrist alarm or a travel clock to remind you when to take them, if you are out of your regular routine. Your cell phone on vibrate can be used if you are in public.

You may need to plan ahead through insurance to get enough medication for a long trip. It's a lot easier to go through your regular routine to pick up your meds and vitamins than to find a drugstore in a strange town, much less abroad. In case your trip is unexpectedly prolonged, carry a clearly written prescription from your doctor, as well as more medication than you think you will need. Keep your medication separate from luggage that could well fly off to another latitude or roll away with someone who has a similar bag.

Make it a practice to carry a written description of your medical problems in your wallet with a list of your medications. It could be useful if you were in an accident. If your RA is severe or you are on a drug that cannot be stopped suddenly, like prednisone, wear a medical alert bracelet or necklace designating your medication, allergies, and other important medical information. (MedicAlert: 800-432-5378 or www.medicalert.) Medic-Alert also has a subscription service that will provide your medical information by phone in case of an accident.

If you carry syringes, you'll need to carry a note from your doctor explaining why you need them. Ask him to specify that they are to be carried on your person, so that they do not end up in Quito when you're in Quebec.

The note is required for flights under the new security rules, as well as at some international border crossings.

Travel insurance

Find out in advance what your medical coverage is when you travel, particularly if you are going abroad. Additional temporary coverage may be a good idea. If you buy a nonrefundable ticket, get trip insurance in case you have a flare and need to cancel.

At the hotel

When you book a room, ask for one near the parking lot and elevators. Ask for the accommodations that you need to be comfortable—a raised toilet seat, grab bars in the bathtub, a bath bench, a nonsmoking room. If there is an exercise room, block out some time in your schedule to use it; there is almost always an exercycle or machine that is easy on your joints. It's less necessary to prod yourself into a hot tub or heated pool, but find out what the amenities are and plan to take advantage of them.

One friend with RA sat in a darkened hotel room, unable to turn the switch with her painful hands, until her husband arrived to turn on the lights. Her solution is to carry an easy-to-turn triangular device that temporarily replaces a dimmer switch.

Cruises

Having backpacked around the world a few times pre-RA, I once turned up my nose at cruise travel. From this point of view, though, it looks like an ideal solution to the need for rest, relaxation, exercise, and adventure. Look into a few things first before you book a trip. Find out the proportion of onboard time to time in port. You may find a lot of land excursions to be wearing, although you can preplan port stays so that you are not on your feet for long hours.

Consider that smaller ships are, well, smaller, and easier to get around. The big ones can be as long as three football fields, but they will have more amenities. Get a floor plan and request a cabin near an elevator or one that is centrally located.

Even if you do not use a wheelchair, you may want to request an accessible cabin. It will be roomier than similarly priced cabins and have bathroom aids such as a raised toilet seat and a shower handrail and seat. Listings of the features in accessible rooms for eleven cruise lines can be found at www.access-able.com (303-232-2979). A letter from your doctor may be required for you to book these rooms, and the availability is limited. If you are having problems walking, you can rent a scooter to take on board (Scootaround, www.scootaround.com, 888-441-7575).

A number of travel agencies specialize in booking travel for people who need special accommodations. You can find one through the American Society of Travel Agents (www.travelsense.org, 703-739-2782). You can find scooter and wheelchair companies at Access-Able Travel (www.access-able.com), but you need to pick through sponsored links for loans and gambling.

Special travel programs

You can probably plan your own best vacation, but it is time-consuming to make arrangements. I do not have a recommendation, but several companies offer packages designed for people with arthritis. Specialized outdoor trips are available from Wilderness Inquiry (www.wildernessinquiry.com). A range of trips, from ancient Cambodian temples to Peruvian wildlife, can be booked through 50Plus Expeditions (www.50plusexpeditions.com). Canyon Ranch Health Resort in Tucson, Arizona, offers a week-long yearly retreat, "Thriving with Arthritis." It includes guidance in exercise, nutrition, and pain management techniques such as meditation, yoga, massage, and relaxation. Support and coping techniques are also offered (www.canyon ranch.com/arthritis).

Elderhostel learning programs, now in ninety countries, are not specifically designed for people with arthritis, but you can choose from a range of physical participation, starting with very moderate. There is also a variety of dietary options. You or your mate need to be over fifty-five to participate. The range of fascinating programs is extraordinary.

Holidays and special events

Holidays, graduations, weddings, showers, anniversaries, birthdays— ordeals to be endured or happy occasions? Planning can make all the difference. For events that are unavoidably lengthy, rest ahead of time and allow time to rest afterward. You are not compelled to do it all. Sometimes the better part of valor is to let others go on with plans if you are risking a flare.

For years I was grinchy about Christmas—not the peace and love and rebirth of Christmas, but the frantic pace, the gift list, the demands beyond my capacity to deliver. Physical and emotional stress increase risk of a flare, so it is no wonder that people with RA often do flare during holidays.

I'll confess, I still face the holidays with trepidation, but I don't end up in a heap any more. When your schedule is interrupted, it's easier to go on tilt, making it much more difficult to take care of yourself. The two most helpful strategies for me have been to stick with my regular routine as much as possible, to share the work, and to simplify. The rhythm of a schedule can carry you through difficult days, so honor its power. Keep your exercise time, your meditation, your time to relax, and allow plenty of sleep.

You can shop online (www.MySimon.com has products from numerous companies). Or print gift certificates for friends—lunch out, for example. Instead of wrapping, use gift bags. You can fill them with colored tissue put through an office shredder. For those gifts you choose to give, many people appreciate a card showing a donation in their name to a cause close to them. There are many. Heifer International offers gifts of animals to people in developing nations—from chicks to buffalo (catalog.heifer.org)—and it is a lot of fun to say you got a goat. Seva can restore a person's sight with cataract surgery in an Asian clinic for forty dollars—a moving gift among others offered at seva.org. You might prefer gifts like this for yourself if someone asks.

The greatest act of simplification for me was deciding that I didn't need to be Uncle Drosselmeyer to everyone. My husband and I abandoned holiday gifts to each other in favor of tokens at birthdays. Drawing names among members of the larger family has relieved a lot of stress and even made the gift hunt fun.

A friend likes to invite people over to trim her tree. Each person has a glass of wassail, and the job is done in good spirit. We fondly remember my mother's friend who showed up with a gift at random times, but never on holidays. It was eccentric, but we took time and pleasure in those gifts. She was a religious person who relished the celebration of holidays without the commercial trappings.

Depression is more prevalent during holidays, so it is important to stay connected with the people with whom you share your life easily.

For a very important event, speak with your doctor about the possibility of rearranging your medications. When I got a cortisone shot as a diagnostic tool, I was told that I could have three more in my lifetime—one for the wedding of each of our sons.

When you are the host

The purpose of getting together is to enjoy your guests, and there are a lot of ways to plan for that. This is the voice of experience speaking: Before you decide to have a houseful, get commitments for help for specific jobs from family or friends. They may be used to being entertained by Superperson.

Think it through. My niece Stephanie once worked for a caterer, and I have learned some tips from her. Take the time to think through how many people can be comfortably accommodated, where they will be located, what furniture needs to be moved or added, what plates and utensils will be needed. Schedule for a time of day when you feel best—brunch, lunch, or dinner. For casual gatherings, telephoned invitations and online e-vites are easy to make. Ask guests to respond so that you can plan food.

Create checklists of all of these things on a clipboard or in a folder. Lay out what you will need ahead of time; Stephanie notes the contents on each serving plate together with serving utensils, which turns out to save a lot of last-minute stress. It gives you time to see if the candle holders are dripped with wax, a platter needs washing, or the ladle is missing.

If you are hosting a meal, it is easier to plan a buffet, letting people serve themselves. Divide preparation over several days, selecting food that can be made in advance, and get help with cleaning. Many guests enjoy participating in last-minute cooking, which provides a chance to visit. People are often glad to bring potluck. Even for big occasions, like Thanksgiving, each family can prepare a dish; we have been doing this for years, and it adds to the convivial tone of the celebration.

You can simplify a casual dinner. Guests can make their own burritos from ingredients you have laid out, dress a baked potato from condiments, or assemble pizzas with store-bought prebaked crusts. A wide selection of prepared foods is available—crudités, prepared lasagna, roasted chicken. Dispense with the cooking altogether by inviting friends over for cards or by renting a movie and picking up takeout. Accept offers for help in cleaning up; it takes only a little effort from several people to dispatch the dishes.

The biggest thing to give up may be your idea of yourself as a great from-scratch cook, if cooking was ever your forte. You can still play in the kitchen as long as you look to your health first. Organizing your time and resources, from work to play, can make it possible for you to continue to do the things you love.

IN A SENTENCE:

> *Organizing your thoughts, time, records, and possessions will help you manage your RA.*

Juvenile Rheumatoid Arthritis

Three types of juvenile rheumatoid arthritis

When Kate Strzok was starting third grade, she took a fall. But the pain in her joints did not go away. Kate, along with three hundred thousand other American children, was diagnosed with juvenile rheumatoid arthritis (JRA), also called juvenile chronic arthritis.

JRA sounds like RA that develops at an early age, but it is actually a name spanning three forms of childhood arthritis that are distinct from the adult form—**polyarticular**, **pauciarticular**, and **systemic JRA**, which is also called Still's disease. Although each is a specific disease, they have some common characteristics: They all involve persistent joint swelling that increases after rest, they more often affect girls, and they may have biochemical similarities.

Kate has polyarticular JRA, which means that it affects more than four joints in a symmetrical pattern. About 30 percent of children with JRA have this form, which usually involves the small joints in the hands and feet. Other joints can be affected, too—for Kate, that means all of them.

Her path through childhood was painful, both physically and emotionally. Most children today can be treated effectively, but that was not true when Kate was diagnosed. She was often not able to attend school because she was stiff until noon, and when her classmates went off to play ball or take dance lessons, she was in the therapy pool at her local hospital. Once wheelchair bound, she is doing well today on one of the new biologic drugs, etanercept, together with methotrexate. Kate is now in college, preparing to study for a year in Rome.

Elise Harris is a typical mischievous four-year-old, except that she has pauciarticular JRA. Half the children with JRA have "pauci." It affects fewer than five joints asymmetrically, typically larger joints, such as the knees. It is not necessarily a lesser disease, because nearly a third of the children with it develop inflammatory eye problems—**iritis** (inflammation of the iris) or **uveitis** (inflammation of the inner eye). Girls under eight years old are most likely to develop this form, and it can begin in infancy.

Elise was seventeen months old when she came down with a persistent high fever, inflamed tonsils, and a progressively inflamed knee. It took four months and 5,400 miles of travel to specialists for her parents to get a diagnosis more specific than "growing pains."

Elise's mother, Misty Harris, was told that the bacterial infection of the tonsillitis had triggered the disease. Elise has uveitis in one eye, and she takes steroid eye drops to control it. Long-term use of steroids can cause cataracts, and Elise is slowly developing one. She takes a low dose of methotrexate to keep the JRA at bay; although liver damage from it is rare, it is also closely watched.

The third type of JRA, systemic onset or Still's disease, accounts for about 20 percent of cases. It can begin suddenly with a fever and a light rash, which may come and go. Inflammation of the joints can spread to internal organs, causing lymph nodes in the neck and other places to swell. The heart can be involved, causing **pericarditis**, and in rare cases, the lungs. A small percentage of these children develop severe arthritis that continues into adulthood.

Medical team

The goals of treatment are to reduce symptoms to promote a normal life for a child and to prevent joint damage. To achieve these goals, all aspects of the disease need to be managed.

The specialists highly trained to deal with the complexities of JRA are pediatric rheumatologists, whose expertise is invaluable. There are, however, few such doctors, and in some areas of the country there are none. (The Arthritis Foundation Web site, www.arthritis.org, provides a link to a directory.) In that case, a pediatrician and a rheumatologist with some experience with children can work in tandem. It took Elise Harris's parents a year and an expedited move from England to start her treatment with a pediatric rheumatologist. At that, they live an hour and a half away.

An ophthalmologist can monitor the risk of eye disease, and an orthopedist can evaluate bone development. An exercise plan can be made by a physical therapist.

Diagnosis

Any kind of JRA is difficult to diagnose. The tests for RA that are, at best, indictors for adults are even more unreliable for children. Because children often compensate for loss of function, they may not complain of pain. Some conditions have similar symptoms, such as physical injury, Lyme disease, infection, malignancies, and other autoimmune diseases. Also, JRA presents differently in each child; it is possible to have a few flares and remission, repeated flares, or a chronic condition.

Various forms of JRA can have similar symptoms; the disease began with a high fever for both Katie and Elise, and both have inflammation of internal organs, which affected Katie's lungs and Elise's eye—although each has a different type of JRA.

A process of elimination is conducted by the physician, using physical examination, medical history, lab tests, and X-rays. JRA is considered after six weeks of chronic joint pain, but it may take longer to come to a diagnosis.

The causes of juvenile arthritis are not known. Some genetic markers are more often found with particular types of JRA and with certain complications, and there may be greater risk within families; still, JRA is not categorized as a hereditary disease.

Lab tests

Although lab tests cannot provide a diagnosis, they may be of help in determining what type of JRA a child has.

Children who are RF positive (rheumatoid factor; see Day 5 for a description of tests) may have a more severe form of polyarticular disease, which is similar to adult rheumatoid arthritis.

Of the children with pauciarticular JRA who have associated eye disease, up to 80 percent test positive for ANA (antinuclear antibody). The disease tends to develop at an early age in these children.

Almost all children with systemic JRA test negative for both RF and ANA.

X-rays can reveal whether or not joint inflammation is the result of injury. It is also used to monitor bone development in children with JRA.

Prognosis

The good news about JRA, according to the National Institute of Arthritis and Musculoskeletal and Skin Disease, is that more than half of affected children outgrow the illness. The prognosis is bright for Elise's joint disease; her doctors think there is a good chance that she will outgrow it, even though her eye will have to be monitored for years after her arthritis is no longer a problem. Kate has not outgrown her arthritis as an adult; however, although she has an occasional flare, it is well controlled.

Although many children with JRA may eventually be symptom free, the disease can affect bone development, resulting in stunted or uneven growth. The use of growth hormones to treat this problem is being explored.

Medications

Any drug for pediatric use has to be tested on children, according to the Pediatric Dosage Equity Act of 2003. A limited number of drugs have been approved for JRA. The law also specifies that child-sized dosage must be designated in prescribing information.

Drugs for children are those that are used for adult arthritis (see Days 6 and 7). They include NSAIDs (nonsteroidal anti-inflammatory drugs) such as ibuprofen and naproxen; DMARDs (disease modifying antirheumatic drugs) such as methotrexate, sulfasalazine, and hydroxychloroquine;

corticosteroids; and BRMs (biologic response modifiers), the new targeted drugs. Some drugs for adults are not FDA approved for use in children.

Methotrexate is often prescribed for children whose symptoms are not relieved by NSAIDs. Patients are regularly screened with blood tests so that the doctor can regulate the dosage to avoid side effects.

Most doctors do not treat children with aspirin because of the possibility that it will cause stomach upset, bleeding problems, liver problems, or Reye's syndrome, a rare brain and liver disease. In some children, however, aspirin in a dosage measured by a blood test can control symptoms.

For severe JRA, corticosteroids (cortisone) may be prescribed to stop such symptoms as inflammation of the sac around the heart. Once the symptoms are controlled, the doctor may reduce the dosage gradually; it is so dangerous to stop suddenly that the taper must be done under medical supervision. Corticosteroids are prescribed with caution in JRA because of negative side effects.

Children with polyarticular JRA may be given a biologic drug that blocks the inflammation-causing protein TNF (see Day 7). Kate Strzok has been taking etanercept (Enbrel), since she was in the original pediatric study, two years before the drug was approved for use in JRA in 1999. Infliximab (Remicade), another biologic TNF blocker, is approved for adults and is being tested on children.

The emotional component

Katie's older brothers protected her from teasing, but they could not prevent the shunning from a best friend who was convinced she was contagious. JRA is not a visible disease, and it can be hard for children to explain.

Almost 20 percent of children experience depression before they are eighteen, and these are kids who don't have JRA to deal with on top of hormones and other vagaries of growing up. It is no wonder that children with JRA can become sad, short-tempered, or withdrawn.

Some research has suggested that symptoms are linked to mood and stress for some children with JRA that interferes with school and social activities. In an effort to understand more about the effects of emotion on these children, The National Institute of Arthritis and Musculoskeletal and Skin Diseases (NIAMS) sponsored a study that followed fifty-one children, from eight to eighteen years old.

The children kept a journal for two months, much like the one described in Week 2. Each day they recorded events and noted the degree to which they were stressful. They also noted arthritis symptoms and whether they had to curtail school or social plans. The children reported symptoms of pain, fatigue, and stiffness on over 70 percent of the days. The journal notes were correlated with physical examinations and lab tests. Elevated stress was related to the days when symptoms increased. Disease activity could be predicted by a change in the level of stress or in mood.

This finding suggests that good medical care needs to go beyond treatment of the physical symptoms of JRA to include management of stress and mood. Cognitive-behavioral therapy was suggested to help improve the emotional development of the children.

Feeling good

Every summer while she was growing up, Katie went to camp MASH (Make Arthritis Stop Hurting) in Wisconsin. She and the other kids, some still her friends, agreed that it was the best week of the year. At camp, she was normal. She didn't have to worry about hurting her hand with a high five. She could put her illness in perspective and learn what to do to get better.

There are ten such camps from Connecticut to Hawaii, as well as other ways to help a child with JRA deal with feelings. Keep communication open. Encourage exercise, which will make her feel better. Be sure that the child does not feel responsible for getting JRA. Join a support group.

Exercise and physical therapy

Exercise plays the same important role in JRA as it does in RA. It is crucial to maintaining muscle tone and range of motion in the joints. Most children can take part in sports when their symptoms are under control. Depending on what joints are involved in a flare, a doctor may change the nature of exercise, but not eliminate it, for the duration. Swimming is especially good, because it uses a wide range of muscles without putting weight on the joints.

A physical therapist can design a program as well as counsel on ways to help guide normal bone growth with splints and other devices.

School

Parents need to advocate for children with JRA at school. It a child's right by law to have an appropriate education, which can be set down in an IEP (Individual Education Plan). Few people understand the nature of arthritis, and so parents can expect to educate the educators about the disease and their child's needs. Design a plan so that flares do not leave the student feeling overwhelmed. Whether it becomes necessary or not, create a fall-back plan, which could involve planning for a tutor, in case the child misses school. Arrange for a set of books to be kept at home, so that they don't need to be carried. Eliminate the joint-stressing backpack in favor of a wheeled pack, as uncool as it is.

Orthotics

Children with JRA can have foot pain that can affect their activities. Shoe inserts are often used to forestall added medication, joint injection, physical therapy, and surgery. A study funded by the Arthritis Foundation set out to discover whether or not that is a good trade.

Researchers divided forty-eight children with JRA who had chronic foot or ankle pain into three groups. They got either new athletic shoes with arch supports and shock-absorbing soles; new shoes with off-the-shelf shoe inserts; or new shoes with custom-made orthotics. Over three months, the children with the custom orthotics had a significant decrease in pain and increase in ability to walk, over the other two groups. The study concluded that correctly fitted custom-made orthotics should be standard in the management of JRA that affects the feet.

Alternative treatments

Many adults with RA seek out alternative treatments. Some, such as relaxation practices, can help a child cope with the stress of a chronic illness. Check with a doctor before adding herbs to a program; some can weaken the efficacy of a drug or even be toxic in combination.

It is important to be alert to the time value of treatment. A detour into an untested remedy may cost more than money. When a child is growing, it is of the utmost importance to control the disease as early as possible.

Research

A national network of pediatric rheumatology centers, the Childhood Arthritis and Rheumatology Research Alliance (CARRA) was established in 2001 in order to coordinate large studies. At this writing, CARRA has been assessing a group of 473 children annually for six to nine years to compare disease progression with medications and lab tests. A new group has been started that will include children who take the new biologic drugs. This data will evaluate long-term outcomes for children with JRA.

A genomics study at Cincinnati Children's Hospital Medical Center is investigating possible genetic causes for JRA. Since 1995, data has been collected on families with more than one child affected by JRA. It has shown that members of the primary family of children with JRA are three times more likely to have an autoimmune disease such as JRA, rheumatoid arthritis, or multiple sclerosis. Other genetic studies have supported the theory that multiple genes are involved in the risk for childhood arthritis. It appears that children with different JRA subtypes have different gene profiles, suggesting that distinct gene combinations are related to different forms of the disease and to degrees of severity.

Making your voice heard

Elise's parents, Misty and Darryl Harris, are on the Arthritis Foundation's Juvenile Arthritis Committee for their region. They are considering working on the national board of that organization, the AJAO (American Juvenile Arthritis Organization, a branch of the Arthritis Foundation) to help spread the word about JRA. The purpose of the boards is to educate and support families affected by the disease. Misty says that privacy protection prevents her from getting the names of new JRA patients, but when she takes Elise to the doctor, she makes the rounds of the waiting room to introduce herself and distribute literature about available support.

The AJAO has a program to encourage more medical students to choose pediatric rheumatology as their specialty. The organization offers to help pay for the extensive and expensive additional training with grants, and programs to forgive loans.

The Harrises are a military family, and with orders to Germany, the search has begun again for expert medical care for Elise, who is thriving.

Katie, too, has a rich and full life. She has no regrets; friends who stayed with her through the hard times are friends for life. There is not much she would change, but she holds out hope for a cure for JRA through stem cell research.

IN A SENTENCE:

> *Juvenile rheumatoid arthritis includes three separate diseases that are treated with adult drugs and additional attention to the physical and psychological growth of children.*

Afterword

HER PORCELAIN skin and billowing red curls take your attention until you see the flicker of a grimace each time she takes a step. Meg has RA, and it has invaded every part of her life. Professional advice and medication are not easy resources for her to access. Unexpected misfortune has left her with neither insurance nor the wherewithal to pay for a doctor or drugs out of pocket.

The competitive system that produces great medical innovations also makes it difficult for many to have them. Managing RA takes tenacity and ingenuity; without money, it takes a great deal more. Meg is not alone in taking a convoluted route through public clinics and Medicare. Most drug companies have created programs to provide prescriptions to those who have no means to get them, like the Encourage Foundation that provides the biologic etanercept.

Not only Meg, but all of us, could be helped by legislation that is slowly wending its way through the Senate (S. 424) and House (H.B. 583) called the Arthritis Prevention, Control, and Cure Act. These bipartisan bills seek to provide additional support to federal, state, and private efforts to prevent and manage arthritis through the National Arthritis Action Plan. Self-management strategies to control symptoms would be taught through a new National Arthritis Education and Outreach Campaign. The legislation will provide expanded support for arthritis research, including JRA, as well as a means to coordinate it through a National Arthritis and Rheumatic Diseases Summit. An education-loan repayment plan is designed to address the shortage of pediatric rheumatologists.

For Meg and for all of us, I encourage you to support this legislation at the Arthritis Foundation Web site, www.arthritis.org; click on Advocacy for updated information and a form letter to sign. Or write directly to your senator or representative.

I leave you in good hands, your own hands, and I wish for you the bountiful life that facing this disease and managing it will bring to you.

Glossary

ADALIMUMAB: Biologic drug with the brand name Humira that targets one of the cytokines that play a role in RA, TNF-alpha. The drug is injected, and approved for adults.

ADRENAL GLANDS: Located above each kidney, the adrenal glands secrete steroid hormones and adrenaline, among other chemicals that help control heart rate, blood pressure, food absorption, and other vital functions that play an important role in stress response.

AEROBIC EXERCISE: Brisk exercise that promotes the circulation of oxygen through the blood. Also called endurance exercise. Examples are running, swimming, and cycling.

AGGLUTINATION TEST: One of two tests for rheumatoid factor (RF), both of which mix a blood sample with antibodies to measure the response.

AMYGDALA: An almond-shaped structure in the brain that integrates the stimuli that evoke fear, triggering a physical stress response.

ANA, ANTINUCLEAR ANTIBODY TEST: A measure of auto-antibodies used in combination with examination, medical history, and other tests in diagnosing RA or determining the type of JRA.

ANAKINRA: A biologic drug, brand name Kineret, that targets the cytokine interleukin-1 (IL-1).

ANALGESICS: A category of pain medications that includes over-the-counter acetaminophen and prescription opiates.

ANTIBODIES: Proteins produced by B cells to fight invading antigens and dispose of them.

ANTIGEN: Anything in the system without a permanent tag that labels it as a "self" cell; a foreign body or organism.

ANTIOXIDANTS: Compounds that help neutralize oxygen-reactive molecules called free radicals that are thought to contribute to disease and tissue damage. Some antioxidants that appear to reduce inflammation are found in fruits and vegetables.

ARAVA: see leflunomide.

ARTHRITIS: A term that includes both osteoarthritis and inflammatory arthritis.

AUTOANTIBODIES: Antibodies, called rheumatoid factor (RF), that target a person's own antibodies as foreign.

B CELLS: Specialized white blood cells, or leukocytes, that operate in the immune response by generating antibodies from the plasma cells they produce.

BMI, BODY MASS INDEX: A number, calculated with height and weight measurements, that indicates whether or not weight is within a healthy range for most people.

BRM, BIOLOGICAL RESPONSE MODIFIERS: New biologic drugs that target specific cytokines active in proliferating autoimmune messages.

CA: Certified acupuncturist.

CAM, COMPLEMENTARY AND ALTERNATIVE MEDICINE: Therapy that is alternative to standard treatment.

CARTILAGE: A thick tissue covering the ends of bones at movable joints which is nourished through the action of exercise. Prolonged inflammation in RA causes damage to cartilage.

CAUDATE NUCLEUS: Tail-shaped masses of gray matter in the brain at the base of each cerebral hemisphere thought to be involved in the reward system as well as in the regulation of voluntary movement.

CBC, COMPLETE BLOOD COUNT: The most common blood test, one of the routine tests advised for regular monitoring of people with RA. It determines the proportions of red and white blood cells and the possibility of anemia.

CHEMICAL SIGNALS: Cell communication throughout the body, conducted by transmission of substances.

CHOLESTEROL: A substance contributing to heart disease, increased by stress.

CHT, CERTIFIED HAND THERAPIST: Occupational therapist with specialized training in caring for elbows, wrists, and hands.

CONSUMERLAB (CL): Provides independent testing of herbs, supplements, and vitamins, with evaluations available online.

CORTICOSTEROIDS: Synthetic drugs closely related to cortisol, a hormone naturally produced in the adrenal gland. Corticosteroids act on the immune system by blocking production of substances that trigger inflammation. Prednisone is the corticosteroid commonly used to treat RA. It does not modify the progression of the disease.

COGNITIVE PSYCHOLOGY: A branch of psychotherapy that addresses the mental processes that underlie behavior and teaches that patterns of thought can be changed.

CORTISOL: A hormone secreted by the adrenal glands. In pregnancy it contributes to an altered immune state, which ensures that the fetus is not rejected as foreign, resulting in temporary remission of RA in the mother.

C-REACTIVE PROTEIN (CRP) TEST: A test, less commonly used than the ESR, used to monitor inflammation in rheumatoid arthritis and other autoimmune conditions. It can be a positive indicator for patients with no detectable rheumatoid factor.

CYCLOOXYGENASE: An enzyme, also called cox, responsible for the production of prostaglandins, intracellular messengers found at high levels in inflammation.

CYTOKINES: Protein chemical messages that regulate gene activity. More than twenty-four different cytokines are thought to play a role in RA. For example, the mix of cytokine messages determines whether T cells will differentiate into cells that promote or diminish inflammation.

DENTAL CARIES: Tooth decay that, in Sjögren's syndrome, can be caused by decreased saliva.

DV, DAILY VALUE: A nutritional reference consolidating previous values with the purpose of decreasing the risk of chronic disease through nutrition.

DMARD, DISEASE-MODIFYING ANTIRHEUMATIC DRUG: A category of drug that influences the progression of RA, including the commonly prescribed methotrexate, as well as biologic drugs.

DOPAMINE: A neurotransmitter associated with elevated feeling. The reward circuits in the brain are rich in dopamine.

DPM, DOCTOR OF PODIATRIC MEDICINE: Podiatrist or foot specialist.

DRI (DIETARY REFERENCE INTAKES): A set of four nutritional reference values that have replaced the 1989 Recommended Dietary Allowances (RDAs): Estimated Average Requirements (EAR), Recommended Dietary Allowances (RDA), Adequate Intakes (AI), and Tolerable Upper Intake Levels, (UL). They are intended to include nutritional levels that can help prevent cardiovascular disease, osteoporosis, certain cancers, and other diet-related diseases.

ENBRIL: Brand name for the biologic drug etanercept.

ENDORPHINS: Proteins naturally produced in the brain that mimic the effects of opiates to block pain by binding to certain neuron receptors. These natural pain blockers are known to be released in the presence of hopeful emotional states.

ENDURANCE EXERCISE: See aerobic exercise.

ESR, ERYTHROCYTE SEDIMENTATION RATE: A test used to measure indicators of inflammation by gauging how quickly red blood cells (erythrocytes) settle in a test tube. Certain proteins present in inflammation adhere to red cells, causing them to stick together and fall more quickly than normal. The rate at which they fall in an hour is the ESR.

ESTROGEN: Female sex hormone. In pregnancy it is one of several hormones contributing to an altered immune state, which ensures that the fetus is not rejected as foreign, resulting in temporary remission of RA in the mother.

ETANERCEPT: Biologic drug that blocks the cytokine or chemical messenger TNF-alpha that plays a role in RA. It is the only biologic approved for use with children.

FIGHT-OR-FLIGHT SYNDROME: The chemical response to stress that, when chronic and unprocessed, can cause health complications.

FLARE: A worsening of inflammation and other symptoms in RA, often connected to stress.

GEL PHENOMENON: Joint stiffness upon waking, a common symptom of RA. The swelling, caused by accumulation of fluid in inflamed tissues, is gradually absorbed back into the blood when joints start moving.

GENETIC MARKER: A recognizable unique location, related to a genetic trait, on a chromosome.

HAQ, THE HEALTH ASSESSMENT QUESTIONNAIRE: The most commonly used patient reporting form for assessing physical function in rheumatoid arthritis trials.

HCT: see hematocrit.

HEMATOCRIT (HCT): A test that measures the volume of red blood cells, given in a number indicating percentage in total volume of blood. A low hematocrit can indicate RA, as well as anemia.

HEMOGLOBIN (HGB): The oxygen-carrying molecule in red blood cells that gives the blood its red color. The test by the same name determines the distribution of oxygen throughout the body and is done as part of the CBC.

HIPPOCAMPUS: An area of the brain known to hold memory, as well as to function in the reward circuits in the brain.

HLA, HUMAN LEUKOCYTE ANTIGEN: A genetic marker composed of proteins found in leukocytes, or white blood cells, that play a role in activating the immune response.

HOMOCYSTEINE: A chemical secreted into the system in response to stress, which increases the risk of heart disease.

HUMIRA: Brand name for the biologic drug adalimumab.

HYDROXYCHLOROQUINE SULFATE, PLAQUENIL: An antimalarial drug containing quinine used for treatment of RA. It is one of the best tolerated DMARDs, although regular eye exams are required.

HYPOTHALAMUS: An area of the brain that stimulates or suppresses release of hormones in the pituitary gland, notably in response to stress, and contributes to control of sleep, body temperature, water retention, appetite, and blood pressure.

IEP (INDIVIDUAL EDUCATION PLAN): A specialized school plan provided for by law for children with special needs. For example, flares in JRA may require a student to have a tutor or extensions on deadlines.

IgG, IMMUNOGLOBULIN G: An antibody that destroys pathogens. In RA, antibodies are produced that identify IgG as foreign, antiself antibodies called Rheumatoid Factor (RF).

IMMUNOGLOBULIN: Antibodies, which are proteins. Each of five classes of immunoglobulin has a different role in the immune response.

INFLAMMATORY ARTHRITIS: A category of arthritis, exclusive of osteoarthritis, that includes infectious arthritis (e.g., Lyme disease) and systemic autoimmune disease (e.g., RA).

INFLIXIMAB: The biologic brand named Remicade that targets the cytokine TNF-alpha. It is infused intravenously.

INTERLEUKIN 1 (IL1): One of the cytokines that play a role in RA, targeted by the biologic drug anakinra (Kineret).

THE IOWA WOMEN'S HEALTH STUDY: Data gathered for half the middle-aged women in Iowa that allows researchers to trace records of those who developed various diseases, including RA. The information is valuable because it is recorded before diagnosis, eliminating recall bias.

ISOMETRIC EXERCISES: Movement that tightens muscles but does not move joints.

ISOTONIC EXERCISES: Moves joints in two phases: concentric, when weight is lifted and the muscles shorten, and eccentric, when weight is lowered more slowly than it would fall, lengthening the muscle.

JUVENILE RHEUMATOID ARTHRITIS (JRA), JUVENILE CHRONIC ARTHRITIS: Three forms of childhood arthritis that are distinct from the adult form: polyarticular, pauciarticular, and systemic JRA, which is also called Still's disease

KINERET: The brand name for the biologic drug anakinra.

LAc: licensed acupuncturist.

LEUKOCYTE: White blood cell or immune cell; there are six types of leukocyte active in the immune system.

LEFLUNOMIDE, ARAVA: A DMARD developed for treating RA. Because the drug may persist for up to two years in the body, it is not appropriate for men or women who may wish to have a child.

LYMPHATIC SYSTEM: The tissues and organs that produce and store leukocytes for fighting infection. They include the bone marrow, spleen, thymus, and lymph nodes—of which there are hundreds: under the arms, in the groin, in the neck.

LPN: Licensed practical nurse. A state-licensed title granted by examination to those who have graduated from an accredited course in practical nursing, a shorter training than that required for registered nurses.

MACROPHAGES: Leukocytes, or white blood cells, that follow the earliest response to infection. They attach to the surface of an antigen to disassemble it and send chemical messages to attract more specialized leukocytes, the B and T cells.

METATARSALS: Five bones in the ball of the foot jointed to the toes in the forefoot and the tarsal bones in the hindfoot. Metatarsal joints are often affected by RA.

METHOTREXATE: The DMARD most often prescribed for RA, originally used for cancer in much higher doses. It works as a decoy, fitting into the same cell receptor as folic acid and diminishing the activity of the immune system. It is often prescribed in combination with a biologic drug.

MFCC OR MFT: Marriage, Family, and Child Counselor, and Marriage and Family Therapist.

MHC, MAJOR HISTOCOMPATIBILITY COMPLEX: Proteins that tag the cells of the body as self cells.

MY PYRAMID: The latest USDA nutrition guideline (www.MyPyramid.com).

NEPHELOMETRY TEST: One of two tests for rheumatoid factor (RF).

NEUTROPHILS: The most common leukocytes (white blood cells) and the first to respond to infection. Billions are produced daily in the bone marrow and live about a day, moving through the system to detect antigens, which they destroy.

NP: Nurse practitioner. A registered nurse with a master's or doctoral degree licensed to diagnose and manage illness, usually in partnership with a doctor. In many states, nurse practitioners are allowed to prescribe medications.

NSAID: Nonsteroidal anti-inflammatory drugs, which are of two types: nonselective NSAIDs include numerous prescription and nonprescription drugs, such as aspirin; selective NSAIDs, cox-2 inhibitors, newer drugs designed to avoid gastrointestinal side effects of nonselective NSAIDs, have been found to have an adverse effect on the heart.

NURSE: RN, LPN, NP; registered nurse, licensed practical nurse, nurse practitioner.

OD: See optometrist (OD).

OPHTHALMOLOGIST (MD): A doctor specializing in the diagnosis and treatment of disorders of the eye, including surgery.

OPTOMETRIST (OD): Doctor of optometry, who prescribes glasses and medications for certain eye diseases.

OSTEOARTHRITIS: A noninflammatory degenerative joint disease generally resulting from wear in older people. It is characterized by joint pain, stiffness, damage to cartilage and bone.

OTR: Occupational therapist.

PANNUS: A sticky deposit of antibodies thickening the lining of the synovium in RA, and stiffening the joint. As the condition improves, the deposit can dissolve.

PAUCIARTICULAR JUVENILE RHEUMATOID ARTHRITIS: One of the three kinds of JRA, in which fewer than five joints, typically larger ones, are asymmetrically affected. Some children develop inflammatory eye problems.

PERICARDITIS: Inflammation of the pericardium, a double membranous sac that envelops and protects the heart.

PHENOTYPE: Disease expression.

PT: Physical therapist.

PLACEBO: A dummy drug, thought to be inert when used as a control in studies. It has since been shown that belief can account for a measurable change in brain chemistry.

PLAQUENIL: See hydroxychloroquine sulfate.

PODIATRIST (DPM): Doctor of Podiatry, foot specialist.

POLYARTICULAR JUVENILE RHEUMATOID ARTHRITIS: One of three types of JRA; it affects more than four joints in a symmetrical pattern.

POLYGENIC SUSCEPTIBILITY: Inclination for a disease to develop under the influence of several genes, each of which alone carries only a small risk. When certain genes occur together in the same individual, the risk for developing RA is increased.

POLYUNSATURATED FATS: Fats recommended to be eaten only rarely because of their association with heart disease, for example, corn, soybean, safflower, and cottonseed oils.

PREFRONTAL CORTEX: An area of the brain involved with the reward circuit, and which is rich in dopamine, a neurotransmitter associated with elevated feeling.

PROGESTIN: A hormone increased in pregnancy and involved with an altered immune state to ensure that the fetus is not rejected as foreign. Progestin prompts the multiplication of regulatory T cells, and may cause remission of RA in the mother that lasts for the duration of the pregnancy.

PROSTAGLANDINS: Hormone-like substances involved in a wide range of body functions, including the inflammation process. Corticosteroids block their production.

PROTEIN-A IMMUNOADSORPTION: A blood filtering process used to treat RA.

PSYCHONEUROIMMUNOLGY: A branch of medicine that studies the relationships of the mind (psycho), the nervous system (neuro), and the immune system (immunology).

PITUITARY GLAND: A small oval-shaped endocrine gland situated at the base of the brain that regulates growth and metabolism. It also plays a role in stimulating the adrenal gland to produce cortisol and adrenaline in the stress response.

PLASMA CELLS: B cells produce antibodies by generating plasma cells—factories that produce about two thousand specific antibodies per second over a few days.

PSYCHOLOGIST: A licensed professional counselor treating personality and cognitive functioning, including adjustment to disability.

PSYCHIATRIST: A medical doctor who specializes in the treatment of mental disorders by therapy that can include medication.

RANGE-OF-MOTION EXERCISE: Activity whose goal is maintaining or improving movement of a specific joint by bringing it through its natural extent of movement.

RDA, RECOMMENDED DIETARY ALLOWANCES: This system of nutritional recommendations, familiar from food labels, is being revised by a system called DRI, Dietary Reference Intakes.

RELAXATION RESPONSE: A deep sense of calm in which blood pressure drops, heart and breathing rate slow, and muscles become less tense. In this state, the body produces more nitric oxide, which is thought to act as an antidote to cortisol and other potentially toxic stress hormones. Developed b yHerbert Benson, MD.

REM SLEEP: Rapid eye movement sleep, a state described as an alert mind in a paralyzed body, characterized by dreaming. It is known to be essential for well-being.

REMICADE: The brand name for the biologic drug infliximab.

REWARD CIRCUIT: The area of the brain that responds to reward stimulus, running from the prefrontal cortex into lower areas including the amygdala and the hippocampus that are rich in dopamine, a neurotransmitter associated with elevated feeling.

RHEUMATOID CACHEXIA: A metabolic change found in rheumatoid arthritis patients accompanied by a loss of muscle, resulting in a lower than normal body cell mass. It has been determined that the condition is a result of lower levels of exercise.

RHEUMATOID FACTOR: Antiself antibodies generated in people with RA that identify some of the body's own antibodies (specifically IgG) as foreign. Many but not all people with the disease test positive for RF.

RHEUMATOID NODULES: Small lumps beneath the skin, about a quarter to half an inch across, developed by some people with RA, often those with more severe disease. These nodules develop from inflammation of a small blood vessel and can appear intermittently. Aside from aesthetics, they do not cause problems.

RN: Registered nurse. A nurse licensed by state examination who has graduated from a nursing program with an associate or bachelor's degree.

SARCOPENIA: Loss of muscle mass through the aging process.

SATURATED FATS: Fats of a type associated with heart disease and recommended to be eaten in small amounts. They are mainly animal fats in whole milk, butter, cheese, and meat, but some are found in plant foods such as coconut oil and palm kernel oil.

SCLERITIS: Inflammation of the whites of the eyes, sometimes a symptom of RA.

SEROTONIN: A hormone and neurotransmitter associated with elevated mood.

SJÖGREN'S SYNDROME: An immunologic disorder that affects moisture-producing glands and occurs in some people with RA, most of them female. The resulting dryness in the eyes, nose, mouth, and vagina needs to be lubricated—in the eyes to prevent damage to the corneas, and in the mouth to prevent dental caries.

STILL'S DISEASE: See systemic onset juvenile rheumatoid arthritis.

STRENGTH TRAINING: Weight-bearing exercise important in RA for building muscle mass to support joints, strengthen the heart and lungs, enhance sleep, and lessen pain, fatigue, inflammation, and stress.

STRESS HORMONE: The hormone cortisol is released in the body in response to stressful environmental stimuli. A chain response, beginning with a chemical signal from the hypothalamus to the pituitary, which then signals the adrenal gland, which results in the release of cortisol to prepare the body for fight or flight.

SULFASALAZINE: A DMARD designed for RA, which appears to help retard progression of the disease, both alone and in combination with other drugs. It includes an antibacterial agent (sulfapyridine) and an anti-inflammatory agent (salicylic acid).

SYNOVIAL JOINTS: The seventy movable joints in the body, which have a joint capsule or cavity containing synovial fluid, a lining of synovial membrane, and cartilage covering the opposing bony surfaces.

SYNOVIAL SAC: The joint capsule or sac lined with a thin membrane, the synovium. The viscous fluid in the sac lubricates the joints and nourishes the cartilage.

SYNOVITUS: A condition in RA in which the synovial sac becomes clogged with immune cells and compounds that fuel inflammation. The joint becomes engorged with new blood vessels and swells.

SYNOVIUM: The thin membrane that lines the synovial sac that encapsulates movable joints. The body's defense system normally enters the joints by way of the synovium, which thickens with excess immune cells in RA.

SYSTEMIC AUTOIMMUNE ARTHRITIS: A category of arthritis that includes rheumatoid arthritis, ankylosing spondylitis, lupus, and gout, among other diverse diseases. It does not include osteoarthritis, which is local rather than systemic.

SYSTEMIC ONSET JUVENILE RHEUMATOID ARTHRITIS: One of three types of JRA, also called Still's disease, characterized by fever, rash, and a possible spread of inflammation to internal organs, causing lymph nodes to swell, and sometimes involving the heart.

SWAN: The Study of Women Across the Nation, a multisite, epidemiologic study of the health of over three thousand women in midlife that examines physical, biological, psychological, and social changes. The study is cosponsored by the

National Institute on Aging (NIA), the National Institute of Nursing Research (NINR), and the National Institutes of Health (NIH), among other agencies.

T CELLS: Specialized leukocytes, or white blood cells, so named because they mature in the thymus. In response to chemical signals, they differentiate into roles that promote or decrease the inflammation causing immune response.

THYMUS GLANDS: Bilateral lymph glands situated under the breast bone, where a new lymphocyte (white blood cell) that has been generated in the bone marrow differentiates into a specialized T cell.

TNF, TNF-ALPHA: Tumor necrosis factor alpha is one of as many as twenty-four different cytokines, or protein chemical messages, that play a role in RA. TNF-alpha is targeted by the biologic drugs adalimumab (Humira), etanercept (Enbrel), and infliximab (Remicade).

TRANS FATS: The fats most closely identified with health problems, usually found in solid form at room temperature, and found most often in fast foods, commercial baking, shortening, and margarine. From partially hydrogenated oil.

TYPE 2 DIABETES: A condition in which production or use of insulin is inhibited, affecting conversion of blood glucose to energy. The same inflammatory chemicals associated with RA can block insulin receptors, raising the risk of type 2 diabetes.

TRIGLYCERIDES: Storage fats, associated with high cholesterol, released in the stress response.

USDA: United States Department of Agriculture, the agency responsible for the dietary guidelines now called My Pyramid.

USP: United States Pharmacopeia, a nonprofit organization that sets standards for drugs and supplements manufactured in the U.S. When a product is tested, the USP mark appears on a label if ingredients stated on the label are present in the declared amount, nutrients are effectively released when it dissolves, and it is free of harmful contaminants. USP does not test for efficacy.

UVEITIS: Inflammation of the inner eye, found in Sjögren's syndrome, an autoimmune condition of the moisture-producing glands, as well as in pauciarticular juvenile rheumatoid arthritis.

VASCULITIS: Inflamed blood vessels.

XYLITOL: A natural sweetener found in plants, fruits, and vegetables, which is also produced in the body by normal metabolism. It has no known toxicity, and is used in products such as syrup, toothpaste, and mouthwash. Xylitol gum is recommended to help produce saliva in a dry mouth, sometimes found in RA patients, to avoid tooth decay.

Resources

WITH THIS book, you begin a lifelong process of learning about your health and about RA. Because changes in rheumatology are coming about so rapidly, you will soon become an old-timer, like me—someone who is keeping up with the breaking news and guiding others.

Finding the information you need can be overwhelming. Narrow it down to trusted sources.

Books about rheumatoid arthritis

The Arthritis Foundation. *Good Living with Rheumatoid Arthritis.* Atlanta: The Arthritis Foundation, 2000.

Lee, Thomas F., Ph.D. *Conquering Rheumatoid Arthritis.* Amherst, NY: Prometheus Books, 2001. Includes a well-presented guide to the immune system in RA.

Imboden, John et al. *Current Rheumatology Diagnosis and Treatment.* New York: McGraw-Hill, 2004. A medical book, intended for physicians.

Koehn, Cheryl et al. *Rheumatoid Arthritis, Plan to Win.* New York: Oxford University Press, 2002.

Lorig, Kate, R.N., Dr.P.H. and James F. Fries, M.D. *The Arthritis Helpbook*. Cambridge, MA: Perseus Books, 2000. This book comes out of the Arthritis Self-Management Program created over twenty-five years ago by Drs. Lorig and Fries. It emphasizes developing self-efficacy skills.

McIlwain, Harris H., M.D., et al., *Winning with Arthritis*. Hoboken, NJ: John Wiley and Sons, 1991.

Nelson, Miriam E. Ph.D. et al. *Strong Men and Women Beat Arthritis*. New York: G.P. Putnam's Sons, 2002. Dr. Nelson has done extensive research at Tufts University and outlines exercise strategies.

Paget, Stephen A., M.D. *The Hospital for Special Surgery Rheumatoid Arthritis Handbook*. Hoboken, NJ: John Wiley and Sons, 2002.

Pisetsky, David S., M.D. *The Duke University Medical Center Book of Arthritis*. Columbine, NY: Fawcett,1991.

Shlotzhauer, Tammi, et al. *Living with Rheumatoid Arthritis*. Baltimore: Johns Hopkins University Press, 2003.

St. Clair, E. William, M.D. et al. *Rheumatoid Arthritis*. Philadelphia: Lippincott, Williams & Wilkins, 2004.

Weinblatt, Michael E., M.D. *The Arthritis Action Program*. New York: Simon & Schuster, 2000. A Harvard Medical School Book.

Related books

Austin, James H., Ph.D. *Zen and the Brain: Towards an Understanding of Meditation and Consciousness*. Boston: MIT Press/USA, 1998.

Cohen, Darlene. *Finding a Joyful Life in the Heart of Pain*. Boston: Shambhala Publications, 2000.

Kabat-Zinn, Jon. *Full Catastrophe Living*. New York: Delta, 1991. One of several books on meditation and mindful living by this writer and seminar leader.

Lewis, Kathleen. *Celebrate Life: New Attitudes for Living with Chronic Illness*. Atlanta: Arthritis Foundation, 2000.

Groopman, Jerome, *The Anatomy of Hope*. New York: Random House, 2004.

Sayce, Valerie, and Ian Frasier. *Exercise Beats Arthritis: An Easy-to-Follow Program of Exercises*. Boulder, CO: Bull Publishing, 1998.

Wells, Susan Milstrey. *A Delicate Balance: Living Successfully with Chronic Illness*, Cambridge, MA: Perseus Books, 2000.

Pamphlets and brochures

At the time of your diagnosis, you may have received a brochure from your doctor published by the Arthritis Foundation. The following can be ordered, a maximum of two at a time, free of charge from the address listed under Organizations below: *Drug Guide, Just Diagnosed, Living with Rheumatoid Arthritis, Make Waves (water exercise), Managing Your Activities, Managing Your Pain, Managing Your Stress, Methotrexate, Rheumatoid Arthritis, Simple Strategies for Change, Supplement and Vitamin Guide, Walking and Rheumatoid Arthritis, When Your Student Has Arthritis.*

From Senior Fitness Productions, 800-306-3137 or www.seniorfitness.com. *Stretching in Bed*, 2001.

From the National Institute of Arthritis and Musculoskeletal and Skin Diseases (NIAMS), Consumer Information Center, www.pueblo.gsa.gov/cic_text/health/rheumatoid;rheumatoid.txt, 877-226-4267.
Handout on Health; Rheumatoid Arthritis.
You can also access the pamphlet at the NIAMS Web site listed below.

Organizations

The Arthritis Foundation
P.O. Box 7669
Atlanta, GA 30357-0669
Toll free phone: 800-283-7800
www.arthritis.org
 Offers a gold mine of arthritis-related information about therapies and lifestyle issues. You can access their regularly updated Web site, which sometimes posts the results of studies. Request free pamphlets from 800-283-7800, order books from 800-207-8633, and request a membership from 800-933-0032. Included with membership is the bimonthly magazine *Arthritis Today*, which can also be accessed online. You can also sign up for periodic e-mail messages called News Alerts.
 The Arthritis Self-Management Program, which promotes self-efficacy, was developed by Kate Lorig, DPH, and James Fries, MD. To locate a course in your area, as well as support groups and other services, enter your zip code at the Arthritis Foundation Web site's Zip Finder. For general questions, call 404-237-8771 or e-mail help@arthritis.org. This national voluntary nonprofit organization funds a wide array of valuable research projects, and deserves your support.

National Institute of Arthritis and Musculoskeletal and Skin Diseases (NIAMS)
National Institutes of Health
1 AMS Circle
Bethesda, MD, 20892-3675
Phone: 301-495-4484
Toll-free phone: 877-22-NIAMS (226-4267)
www.nih.gov/niams
   Provides regularly updated information about various forms of arthritis, distributes
   educational materials, and lists links to other sources of information.

Missouri Arthritis Rehabilitation Research and Training Center
1 Hospital Drive
Columbia, MO 65212
Toll-free phone: 877-882-6826
www.muhealth.org/arthritis
   The only federally funded arthritis rehabilitation research and training center;
   resources are available through the Web site.

The American College of Rheumatology
1800 Century Place, Suite 250
Atlanta, GA 30345
Phone: 404-633-3777
Fax: 404-633-1870
www.rheumatology.org
   Professional nonprofit organization based in Atlanta, for rheumatologists and
   associated health professionals. Develops treatment guidelines. Directory of
   rheumatologists is by no means complete.

Health newsletters

Nutrition Action Health Letter
1875 Connecticut Ave., N.W., Suite 300
Washington, D.C., 20009-5728
www.cspinet.org
   The largest-circulation health newsletter in North America is Nutrition Action Health
   Letter, published by Center for Science in the Public Interest for over thirty years.
   C.S.P.I. is an independent nonprofit consumer health group that accepts no
   government or industry funding. Their well-researched and -presented newsletter,
   which covers much more than food, is available by subscription. You can sign up on
   their Web site.

There are several good ones from universities:

Harvard Medical School: *Harvard Health Letter, Women's Health Watch, Men's Health
Watch, Heart Letter, Mental Health Letter*, www.health.harvard.edu, each with
subscriptions that give access to archives. Books are also available to buy as print or
downloads.

Tufts University Health and Nutrition Newsletter, www.healthletter.tufts.

University of California: *The Berkeley Wellness Newsletter*, subscription gives access to archives; www.wellnessletter.com.

Internet resources

The Internet is a mixed blessing. Anyone can put up a site, and anyone does; the Net is full of opportunists wanting to sell you arthritis potions that will have you in toe shoes by the next morning. Web sites change frequently and bona fide sites can be linked to sham sites. Managing this disease is work, fatigue can dull acuity, and it can be tempting to believe the unbelievable. Be careful out there in cyberspace. The upside of the blessing is that the Net has excellent resources for RA, and the most recent information.

If you have not grown up with the Internet, it's well worth venturing into it. Most public libraries have free access. The suffix on a web address indicates its category:

○ .com—a commercial site that is selling something
○ .org—an organization such as the Arthritis Foundation
○ .gov—a government Web site
○ .edu—a site at an educational institution

Medical dictionaries: I suggest that you bookmark, or save a connection to, an online medical dictionary, particularly if you are reading professional studies. Medline Plus, the dictionary site offered by the National Institutes of Health, www.nlm.nih,gov/medlineplus/mplusdictionary.html, is my first choice of several. Words in the definition can be further defined at the site. On the occasions when Medline is too technical, you can key into your search engine "what is" followed by the word you want defined.

The American College of Rheumatology (ACR) lists the diagnostic criteria for RA that they have established: www.rheumatology.org.

Arthritis, Rheumatism, and Aging Medical Information System (ARAMIS), Department of Immunology and Rheumatology, Stanford University Department of Medicine, www.aramisstanford.edu, where you will find the Health Assessment Questionnaire.

The European League against Rheumatism posts the research papers presented at a yearly international symposium at www.EULAR.org.

Nancy Etchemendy's Web site, The Rheumatoid Arthritis Hope Page: www.sff.net/people/etchemendy/arthritis. A recognized children's writer who has had RA for decades posts her experiences.

The Mayo Clinic Web site, www.MayoClinic.com, has RA information, including recommended exercise and alternative treatments.

Monterey Bay Aquarium Seafood Watch lists fish known to contain toxic chemicals, as well as endangered species (www.mbayaq.org and click seafood watch).

The National Library of Medicine offers abstracts of articles at the Medline site, www.nlm.nih.gov. For an entire article, contact the medical journal to order a reprint or go to a medical library; a teaching university will have an extensive collection of medical journals.

Forums

A forum is an online meeting place devoted to a common topic where people can communicate either in real time by typing messages and responses, or by posting on a bulletin board to gather comments at a later time. Regardless of which Internet service provider you use, you can network through these forums.

Access the chat room on About.com by searching for Carol Eustice's site. You will find the link at the lower left corner. You will need to register with a member name, by which you will be addressed by others in the chat room, and password. It is open for two hours each evening and frequented by some people who have long experience with RA and related diseases, as well as those who are newly diagnosed.

An interactive bulletin board on RA can be found at www.arthritis insight.com.

Med Help International site: At the Rheumatology page, posted questions are answered by Dr. Kevin Pho, www.medhelp.org/forums/Arthritis/wwwboard.html.

Nutrition

American Dietetic Association consumer nutrition hotline, 800-366-1655, www.eatright.org.

Consumer Lab tests supplements to determine if they are accurately labeled and the contents are both safe and in an absorbable form. There is information available without charge, as well as access to studies through paid membership: www.ConsumerLab.com.

Food and Nutrition Information Center, National Agriculture Laboratory, USDA, www.fns.usda.gov/fns.

Healthfinder-Gateway to Reliable Consumer Health Information, US Department of Health and Human Services, www.healthfinder.gov.

National Institutes of Health, Office of Dietary Supplements (ODS), www.dietary -supplements.info.nih.gov, and www.cc.nih.gov/ccc/supplements/intor.html.

United States Pharmacopeia sets standards for toxic chemicals in supplements: www.usp.org lists approved products.

USDA nutritional information: www.pueblo.gsa.gov and www.mypyramid.com.

Exercise

The Arthritis Foundation sponsors the following exercise courses and programs: Walk with Ease, PACE (People with Arthritis Can Exercise), and the Arthritis Foundation Aquatic Program. PEP. Books and videos of these programs are available from the Arthritis Foundation, 800-933-0032, or borrowed from individual chapters: www.arthritis.org.

BMI, body mass index: The National Institutes of Health (NIH) National Heart, Lung and Blood Institute site will automatically calculate your BMI when you enter your height and weight: http://nhlbisupport.com/bmi/bmicalc.htm. Another site has a chart for finding your BMI: *Body Mass Index (BMI) Chart.*

Pedometers: Pick up an inexpensive one up at a sporting goods store. You won't need special added gizmos unless you want to pay more: Yamax Digi-Walker, www.digiwalker.com; New-Lifestyles, 888-748-5377, www.new-lifestyles.com; SportLine Electronic Pedometer, 914-964-5200, www.sportlline.com.

Tufts University and the Center for Disease Control have created an animated exercise program at http://nutrition.tufts.edu/research/growingstronger/. You can download a 116-page book of exercises at this site, *Growing Stronger; Strength Training for Older Adults.* Also see the book by Dr. Miriam Nelson of Tufts, one of several listed above.

The University of Missouri Arthritis Rehabilitation Research and Training Center has produced the Good Moves for Every Body Exercise Video, available from www.hsc.missouri.edu.

Aids

Be attentive when going onto Web sites for aids. There is a mixed bag of products. Together with a useful jar opener, you can find a book promoting a crackpot diet and a pricey curative cream with ingredients you could buy in the drugstore under another name for a fraction of the cost and none of the hype.

The Arthritis Foundation Ease of Use program tests product in a lab to determine their joint-friendliness. For a list of products that have been recognized by Ease of Use, see www.arthritis.org.

Aids for Arthritis, Inc.
35 Wakefield Drive
Medford, N.J.
Toll-free phone: 800-654-0707
www.aidsforarthritis.com
　　Aids for Arthritis has an online catalog of aids for the kitchen, dressing, bathing.

For the office:

Egonomic Solutions
129 N. Sylvan Drive
Mundelein, IL 60060-4949
Toll-free phone: 800-755-4950
www.goergo.com
　　Arm supports, copy holders, keyboards, and other office innovations are offered here. Other sources for a computer mouse designed to take the strain off the hand: Virtually Hands Free computer mouse, Designer Appliances, www.aerobicmouse.com. Cirque Cruise Cat, a touchpad device that moves the cursor: www.cirque.com.

Desk aids:

Pilot brand Dr. Grip pens and pencils, Fiskers Softouch scissors.

Preprinted journals:

Memory Minder—Health Journal, Exercise Journal, or Diet Journal, www.Memoryminded.com

Personal items:

Shoe inserts: First check out your drugstore, and also consider custom orthotics. Cushioned antipronation inserts (CAPI) come in various thicknesses, 800-643-5536, www.shoeinserts.com. Dr. Scholl's Tri-comfort Orthotics are found at most drugstores, www.drugstore.com. SoftSole Performance Graphite Orthotics are available online and at retail outlets: www.sofsole.com. Sorbothane's SorboGel Insole, 877- 797-6726 www.rxsorbo.com. Spenco PolySorb Inserts, www.thesportsauthority.com.

Speed Strap substitute for shoelaces: www.speedstrap.com.

Clothing—well designed, easy to put on, wrinkle resistant or wash and wear, designed for travelers and those who don't like to iron: Easy Does It, www.myeasydoesit.com. Chico's, 888-855-4986, www.chicos.com. Spiegel, 800-435-4500, www.spiegel.com. Eddie Bauer, 800-625-7935 www.eddiebauer.com.

Keyring: Orbit key ring, www.solutionscatalog.com enables you to remove or add keys by pressing a stainless steel ball.

At home:

Oxo kitchen tools, www.Oxo.com; 800-545-4411—large-handled tools such as a soap-dispensing scrub brush, vegetable brush, whisk, peeler, ice cream scoop. A slicer called a mandoline allows almost horizontal motion.

Peta Easi-grip tools. An American Web site for a British company with well-designed hand tools: www.peta-uk.com/usashop.

Organizing: A number of organizing books and Web sites are full of good ideas; www.flylady.net has suggestions on keeping a home in order.

Solar cookers: www.solarcookers.org, or www.solarovens.org

Juvenile Rheumatoid Arthritis

The Juvenile Arthritis Foundation
American Juvenile Arthritis Organization
1330 West Peachtree Street
Atlanta, GA 30309
Phone: 404-872-7100
Toll-free phone: 800-283-7800
www.arthritis.org
> Part of the National Arthritis Foundation, this organization is a nonprofit group devoted to childhood rheumatic diseases. It has information about JRA, support groups, and pediatric rheumatology centers around the country.

Kids on the Block, Inc.
9385-C Gerwig Lane
Columbia, MD 21046
Phone: 410-290-9095
Toll-free phone: 800-368-KIDS (5437)
www.kotb.com
> An educational program that uses puppets to show how JRA can affect school, sports, friends, and family. A package of puppets and scripts is available for a fee.

Alternative resources

BIOFEEDBACK

Biofeedback Certification Institute of America, www.bcia.org, lists some certified practitioners by area.

ACUPUNCTURE

For a list of certified acupuncturists, American Association of Acupuncture and Oriental Medicine at 888-500-7999 or www.aaom.org as well as www.acufinder.com. For a medical doctor trained to do acupuncture, American Academy of Medical Acupuncture, 800-521-2262, www.medical acupuncture.org.

The National Center for Complementary and Alternative Medicine web site: http://nccam.nih.gov.

Drugs

Keep track of new medications approved by the FDA by subscribing to the FDA-Druginfo List at www.fda.gov. At this site there is also information on clinical trials and how they are conducted.

National Institutes of Health site lists clinical trials for RA by area at www.clinicaltrials.gov.

The makers of the new biologic drugs have Web sites and offer toll-free numbers for inquiries:

Enbrel: patient support line, 888-546-3738; educational program called Enliven, and a Web site, www.enbrel.com. There is an educational program called RA Access, 800-395-2270; www.ra-access.com.

Kineret: customer support line, 866-546-3738; Web site www.kineretrx.com.

For Remicade: information line, 886-736-4273; Web site www.remicade.com.

To dispose of unused medications if you do not have a hazardous waste center nearby, call 800-CLEANUP (800-253-2687) or log onto www.1800cleanup.org. For used sharps, ask the pharmacist where you buy them for the nearest depository, usually at a hospital or pharmacy. You will receive an empty sharps container in exchange for the one you bring in; I use several to minimize trips.

Acknowledgments

WHY IS the vocabulary of gratitude so sparse compared to that of despair? Perhaps it is closer to the wordless center of the heart. I can show it with my hands, though, no small accomplishment for some with RA—putting my palms together and touching my forehead, pumping a fist in the air.

For guiding me through the most desperate of times, thank you seems a small thing to say to Dr. Kenneth Sack of the University of California at San Francisco. I am grateful for who he is, a compassionate physician who spreads hope, and for what he knows, a wise professor of rheumatology. His reply, when I asked him for a watchword for the writing of this book, is posted above my computer: "Be humble. Ken Sack." That is, I observe, his own governing maxim.

Thanks to my cousin, Dr. Daniel McNeil, a podiatrist who was the first to suggest my diagnosis from another state without seeing me, and for his willingness to share his expertise. Thanks to Dr. Mel Britton for opening his office alone on a Sunday to confirm my diagnosis. And thanks to the staff at the Arthritis

Clinical Trials Center at UCSF, especially to Steve, who examined each of my joints for two years in the trial of a new biologic drug.

The contribution to this book by Dr. Lindsey Criswell, who heads the UCSF Rheumatoid Arthritis Genetics Research Unit has been generous and invaluable. I also appreciate the contribution of Dr. David Wofsy, George A. Zimmerman Distinguished Professor of Rheumatology at UCSF, on biologic drugs.

Thanks to writers Sarah Wilson and Nancy Etchemendy, whose decades of experience with RA have informed both this book and my life. They are as innovative at living with this chronic disease as they are at creating the children's literature for which they have each been so richly recognized.

Kate Strzok and Misty Harris exemplify the way I hope this book can teach one to face arthritis. Kate told me her own story, straightforward through the hard times, without regret. I would wish for all children with JRA a parent like Misty Harris, who has been willing to go anywhere and do anything for her daughter, holding out a hand to others along the way. And thanks to all those with RA to whom I have spoken, both in person and online, to gather material for this book.

Thanks to those writers who read chapters and offered guidance: Esther Baron, Geraldine Lanier, Genna Panzarella, Heather Preston, Marty Rice, Dorothy Slate.

Particular thanks to Sue Severin for reading the manuscript. Once her college teaching assistant, I was grateful to again benefit from her careful eye.

I would like to acknowledge Howard Grossman for the cover design and Pauline Neuwirth, who designed the interior pages of the book.

A special note of gratitude to Suzanne McCloskey, my editor, for kind words that warmed me and fueled this writing. And thanks as well to assistant editor Peter Jacoby for assistance large and small.

My husband, Jerry Draper, has made this book possible in every way.

Index